At the core of your body's complex blood-filtering an waste removal systems, the Kidneys and Bladder get **clogged, attacked** and **mutilated** by the constant barage of toxic chemicals and pollutants found everywhere in modern society.

Cleansing, purifying and **detoxifying** the Kidneys and Bladder on an annual basis is the **ONLY** way to keep them functioning according to God's Plan.

DR. RICHARD SCHULZE TEACHES YOU HOW!

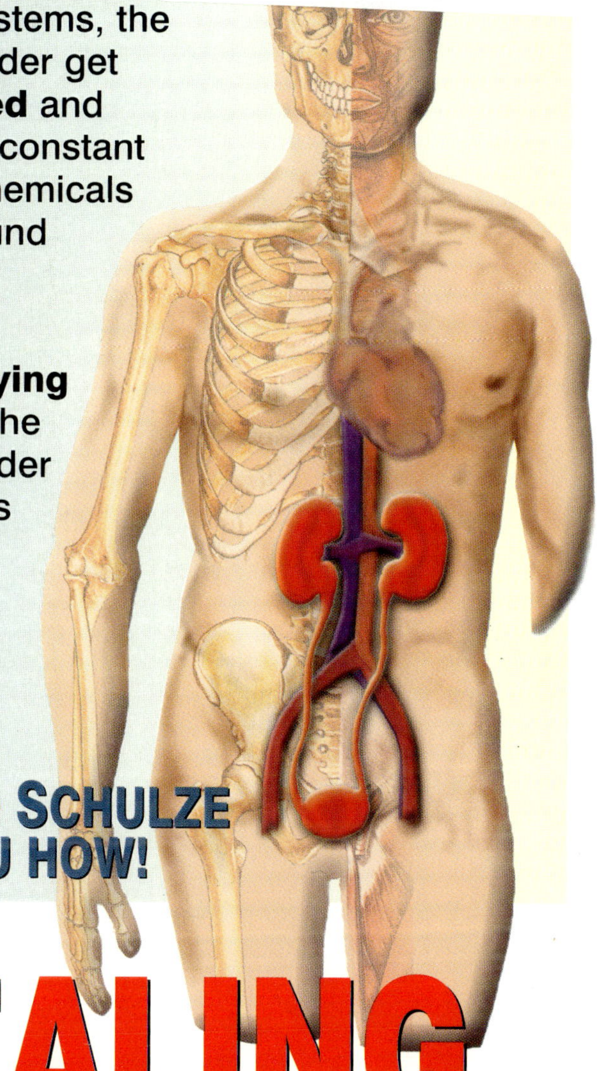

HEALING
KIDNEY & BLADDER DISEASE
NATURALLY

NATURAL HEALING PUBLICATIONS

Published by Natural Healing Publications
P.O. Box 9459, Marina del Rey, California 90295
1-877-TEACH-ME (832-2463)

Library of Congress Catalog Card Number: PENDING
Healing Kidney and Bladder Disease Naturally

ISBN: 0-9671567-8-5

PRINTED IN THE USA ON 100% CHLORINE AND BLEACH-FREE RECYCLED PAPER, WITH MINIMUM 50% POST-CONSUMER WASTE (REALLY RECYCLED WASTE) USING SOY-BASED INK.

WARNING!

A WARNING from our Lawyers:

This book is published under the First Amendment of the United States Constitution, which grants the right to discuss openly and freely all matters of public concern and to express viewpoints no matter how controversial or unaccepted they may be. However, Medical groups and Pharmaceutical companies have finally infiltrated and violated our sacred Constitution. Therefore we are forced to give you the following WARNINGS:

If you are ill or have been diagnosed with any disease, please consult a medical doctor before attempting any natural healing program.

Many foods, herbs or other natural substances can occasionally have dangerous allergic reactions or side effects in some people. People have even died from allergic reactions to peanuts and strawberries.

Any one of the programs in this book could be potentially dangerous, even lethal, especially if you are seriously ill. Therefore, any natural method you learn about in this book may cause harm, instead of the benefit you seek.

ASK YOUR DOCTOR FIRST, but remember that the vast majority of doctors have no education in natural healing methods and herbal medicine. They will probably discourage you from trying any of the programs in this book.

TABLE OF CONTENTS

TABLE OF CONTENTS

FOREWORD

Assimilate and Eliminate

The *OLD IN* and *OUT*

You and every organ in your body, in fact every one of your 100 trillion cells, have the same two basic functions – In and Out, In and Out, In and Out. ***Assimilate*** nutrition **in** and ***Eliminate*** waste **out.** And, when it comes to the out (the elimination of waste), your body only has two major ways to get this waste out of your body. Your *solid* waste is removed by your Large Intestine and your *liquid* waste is removed by your **Kidneys and Bladder.**

Your solid waste removal system, your intestinal tract, is as long as two cars parked end to end. It is a big, long tube from your mouth to your anus. Just part of this system, your colon, is the biggest organ in your body, measuring in at 7 inches in circumference and 60 inches long.

On the other hand your Kidneys are much more refined organs. They are comprised of approximately two million very complex, microscopic units called Nephrons that filter mostly liquid waste out of your blood. This end waste product is called urine and is about 95% liquid and 5% dissolved substances like minerals, nitrogen waste products and even blood, pus, bacteria, and microscopic parasites.

As I always say, on a very gross level, scientists and medical doctors understand the *basic* anatomy and physiology of the urinary tract, in other words the *basic* parts and how they work. But this system, as you will see me describe in Chapter 2, like all systems of the human body, is really beyond mankind's comprehension.

Early on in my medical career it became very obvious to me that the human body was designed and put together by someone or some force much greater and much smarter than me. Therefore, the next simple, logical and common sense conclusion for me to make, was to never attempt to heal this amazing machine from the *inside,* like medical doctors do with surgery, radiation, chemotherapy and even Kidney Transplants, but instead to heal the human body from the outside by creating a healthy lifestyle – **STOPPING** my patients from doing what made them sick and what hurt their organs in the first place and **STARTING** them on new habits that healed the bodies and prevented future disease, this is what created the thousands of healing miracles in my clinic.

In this book I will take you on a journey. In the first chapter, I will expose just how bad the Kidney and Bladder disease *epidemic* has gotten in America, from the over 40 Million Americans with Kidney impairment, infections and disease to the 100,000 new cases of Kidney and Bladder cancer every year to the skyrocketing sales increases of adult diapers.

Then, as usual, in the second chapter I will simplify the Kidneys, the Bladder and the entire Urinary System so anyone can understand it. At least you will know the basic parts and the fundamental ways it works which can help when you, a loved one, or a friend gets sick. More importantly, this information can help you get well.

In the third chapter, I tell you all about Kidney and Bladder disease with lots of pictures that will hopefully shock you and motivate you into the fourth chapter, which includes my many ***natural*** flushes, routines and programs that I developed in my clinic which will help you clean, detoxify, strengthen and protect your Kidneys and Bladder.

Friends, don't be the Average American. Don't suffer with painful and debilitating diseases and destroy and shorten your life. Don't be like the Average American and torture yourself with the horror, pain and bankrupting expense of medical doctors, hospitals and drugs.

Healing yourself of anything is easy, simple and your God-given right. Your body knows how to heal you of anything, any disease. It has the blueprint, the plans and all it needs is your assistance.

The very easy and simple programs in this book can change your life. As I always say, a little knowledge is a powerful healing tool.

Stay Healthy, Enjoy Life and Have Fun.

Dr. Richard Schulze

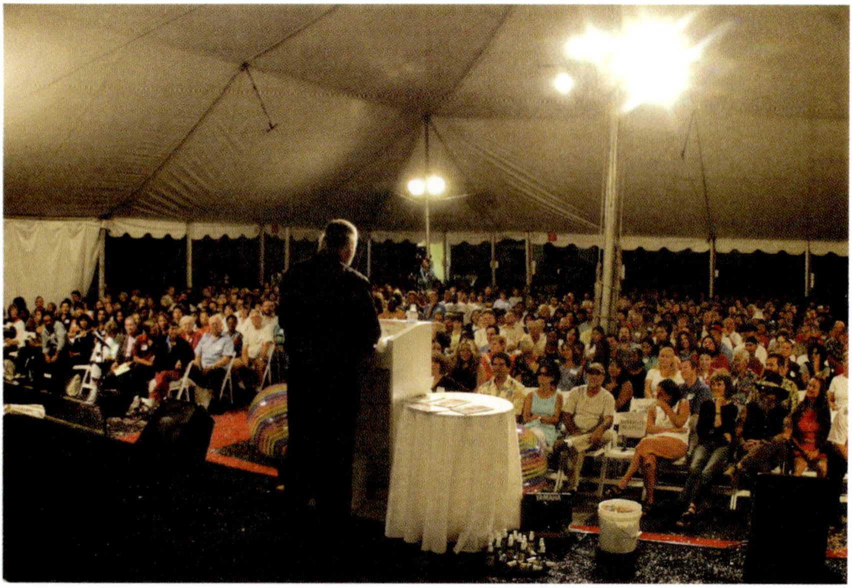

"I have never healed anyone of any disease. On the contrary, I have* taught *a lot of people how to heal themselves. After all, the word doctor originates from the old Latin word,* docere*, which literally means* to teach. *Over the years, many of my patients referred to me as their teacher or guru, instead of their doctor. I always liked that because, after all, not much teaching takes place in a hospital emergency room."

– Dr. Richard Schulze

"The doctor of the future will give no medicine, but instead will interest their patients in the care of the human frame through lifestyle and diet, and in the cause and prevention of disease."

– Thomas Edison, 1847-1931

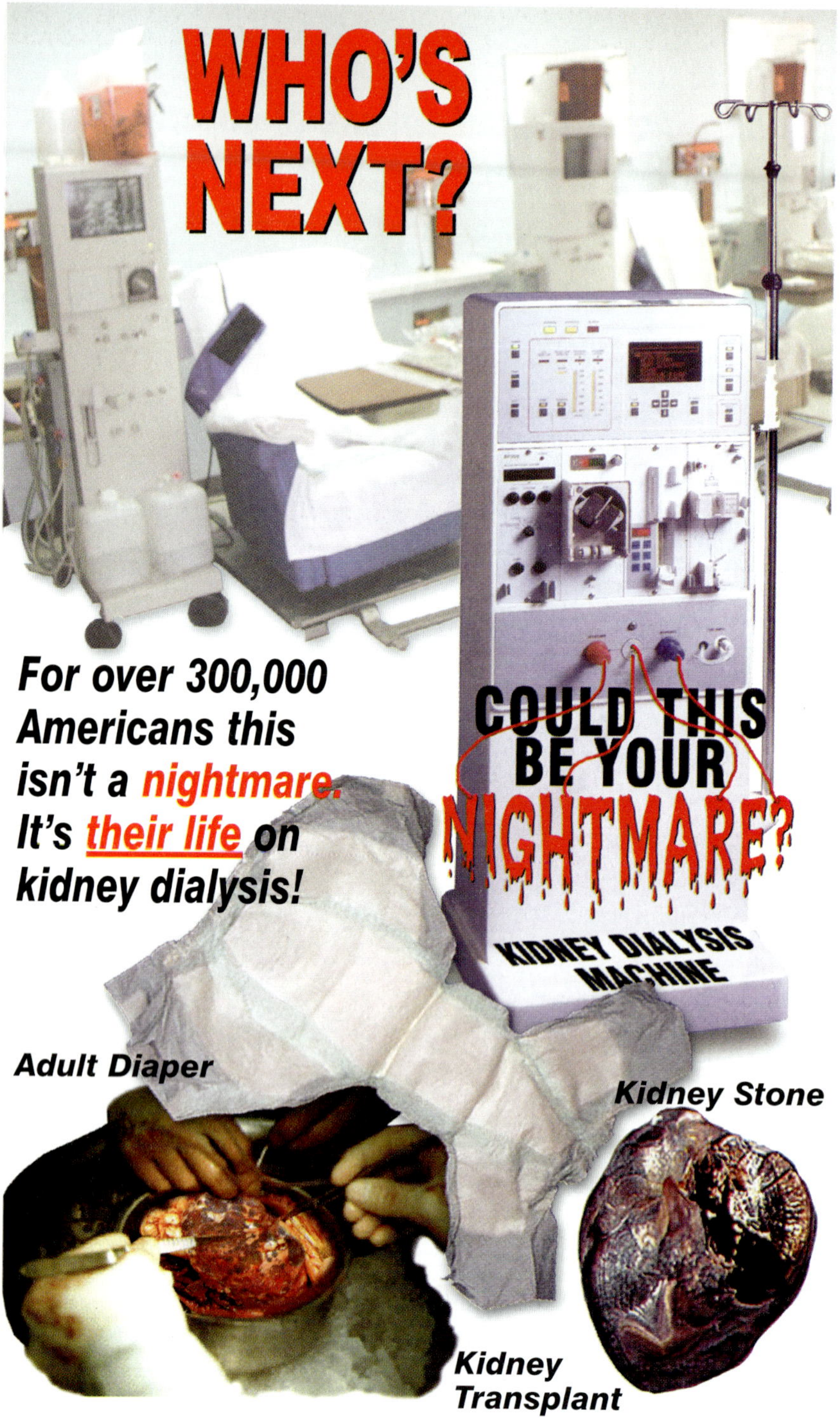
WHO'S NEXT?
For over 300,000 Americans this isn't a nightmare. It's their life on kidney dialysis!
COULD THIS BE YOUR NIGHTMARE?
KIDNEY DIALYSIS MACHINE
Adult Diaper
Kidney Stone
Kidney Transplant

CHAPTER ONE

Kidney and Bladder Disease – The PREVENTABLE EPIDEMIC

FACTS

Over 300,000 Americans DRAIN THEIR BLOOD with dialysis mechanical vampires.

Over 40 MILLION Americans have Kidney & Bladder INFECTIONS, IMPAIRMENTS AND DISEASE.

INCONTINENCE – The *New* American epidemic attacks over 20 MILLION Adults.

Kidney and Bladder CANCER attacks over 90,000 Americans.

"It's so silly that Kidney and Bladder Disease has become an epidemic in America, especially since it's so easy to prevent . . . and so simple to heal."

There is nothing more debilitating and horrifying than Kidney and Bladder disease. Just imagine having your veins punctured and hooked up through plastic tubes to a machine that drains every drop of blood out of your body because your kidneys are too degenerated to filter it themselves. You feel horrible and weak because your blood is critically overloaded with toxic waste and poison. If you don't have it drained out you will die. This is like a recurring vampire nightmare that keeps playing over and over again, but you can't wake up because . . . . you are awake!

FACT: ***The American Society of Nephrology reports that***

OVER 40 MILLION AMERICANS HAVE KIDNEY AND BLADDER INFECTIONS, IMPAIRMENT AND DISEASE

THE SOLUTION – it's very simple. Effective Natural Healing Programs and Powerful Herbal Formulae can stop Kidney and Bladder Disease right in its tracks. **Chronic Kidney Disease often starts with a Kidney or Bladder infection, and because many are asymptomatic, many people don't even know they have one.** This is why my routine 5-Day Kidney/Bladder Cleansing and Detoxification Program with Kidney and Bladder ***FLUSHING*** drink was a standard ***yearly*** protocol for ALL of my patients in my clinic. Also, every patient that came to see me with a Kidney and Bladder Infection healed it using herbs. **EVERY ONE OF THEM, NO EXCEPTIONS, 100%.** For over 20 years I saw Kidney and Bladder herbs destroy every type of infection in the Urinary tract.

In fact, I still have audio tapes from my clinic answering machine with patients exclaiming their shock and surprise that my herbal formulae "did what no medical doctor and no antibiotic could do," which was cure their chronic Kidney and Bladder infections.

These same herbs I discuss in this book are so powerful they are now listed in the Merck Index, a leading medical chemistry book published by a drug manufacturer, as diuretics and urinary antiseptics.

FACT: INCONTINENCE – THE *NEW* AMERICAN EPIDEMIC ATTACKS OVER 20 MILLION ADULTS.

I had a female patient named Joan who was about 50 when she came to see me. Her life had been devastated, literally ruined with over 20 years of incontinence. This poor woman had no life, her husband divorced her, she didn't have any social life, she lived in adult diapers and rushed home every day after work to hide in her apartment, covered with urine. She hadn't had a date nor made love in 15 years.

Kimberly-Clark reports sales of their Depends adult diapers has skyrocketed increasing 85% in just the last few years.

The medical doctors said that there was nothing that could be done. What they should have told Joan was that there was nothing *(that THEY knew of)* that could be done. After just a few months of simple lifestyle changes and my Kidney and Bladder Programs her incontinence was subsiding and she started going out, dating and even started taking ballroom dancing lessons. I didn't see her for a few months and then all of a sudden I got a postcard through my clinic mail slot from her. She was in Europe ***CLIMBING THE MATTERHORN WITH HER NEW HUSBAND!!!*** **So much for *incurable!***

FACT: KIDNEY AND BLADDER CANCER ATTACKS OVER 90,000 A YEAR.

Undetected and untreated Kidney and Bladder Infections are most often the beginning of organ scarring, degeneration and cellular breakdown. Eventually you get Kidney failure and all too often. . . Cancer, which eats you alive from your urinary tract out. This is so unnecessary because it is so easy to prevent. Not only because Kidney and Bladder Infections are 100% curable as I mentioned on the cover, but also because it is a common medical fact that if you make sure that you drink only 2 quarts of liquid a day (water, fresh juice and herb tea),you *REDUCE* your risk of developing Kidney and Bladder cancer by 50%. That's right, you heard it right, **drinking more water PREVENTS Kidney and Bladder Cancer!**

The reason for this is very simple. There are many potentially carcinogenic (cancer causing) toxic chemicals and waste materials found in the urine. **If you drink less liquid, your urine is more concentrated and also flows less frequently.** This longer exposure time of concentrated urine against the delicate inner tissues of your bladder increases irritation, infection and eventually Cancer. Drinking more liquid, especially water, juice and herb tea, dilutes these poisons in your urine and also creates more urine flow which in turn reduces the exposure time these potentially carcinogenic chemicals have in your bladder. In other studies just one glass of high quality cranberry juice was found to reduce bladder infections by 80%.

Sure, as usual, modern medicine is ignorant of simple healthy living and lifestyle changes that can prevent Kidney and Bladder Disease, and heal it too. Medical doctors and hospitals can make a lot more money treating Urinary Disease with the dialysis machine pictured here, at a cost of about $75,000.00 a year per person on average.

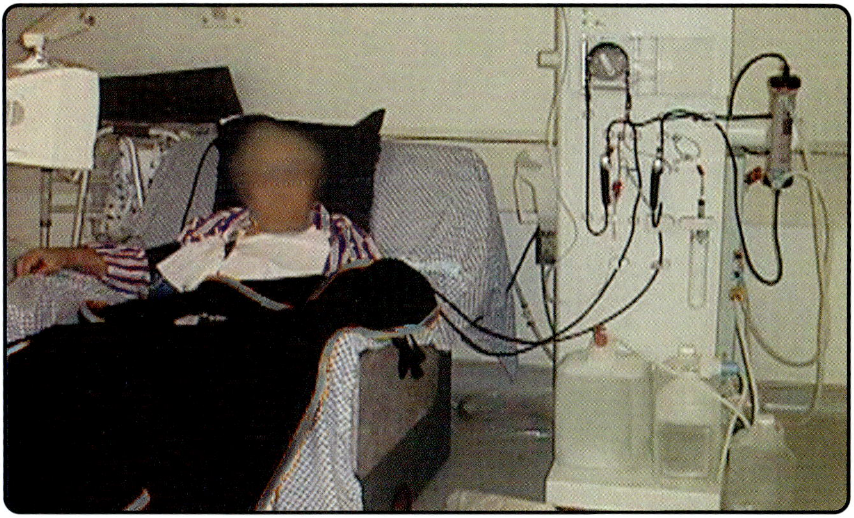

Remember the old medical credo, the hippo***critic*** oath, ***a patient healed is money lost. So Friends,***

PLEASE, PLEASE, PLEASE

protect yourself by preventing Kidney and Bladder Disease, in this case just a few more ounces of water is worth a pound of cure.

However, if you already suffer from ANY Kidney or Bladder infection or disease START NOW on my 5-Day Kidney/Bladder Cleansing and Detoxification Program outlined in Chapter Five of this book.

THE URINARY SYSTEM *SIMPLIFIED*

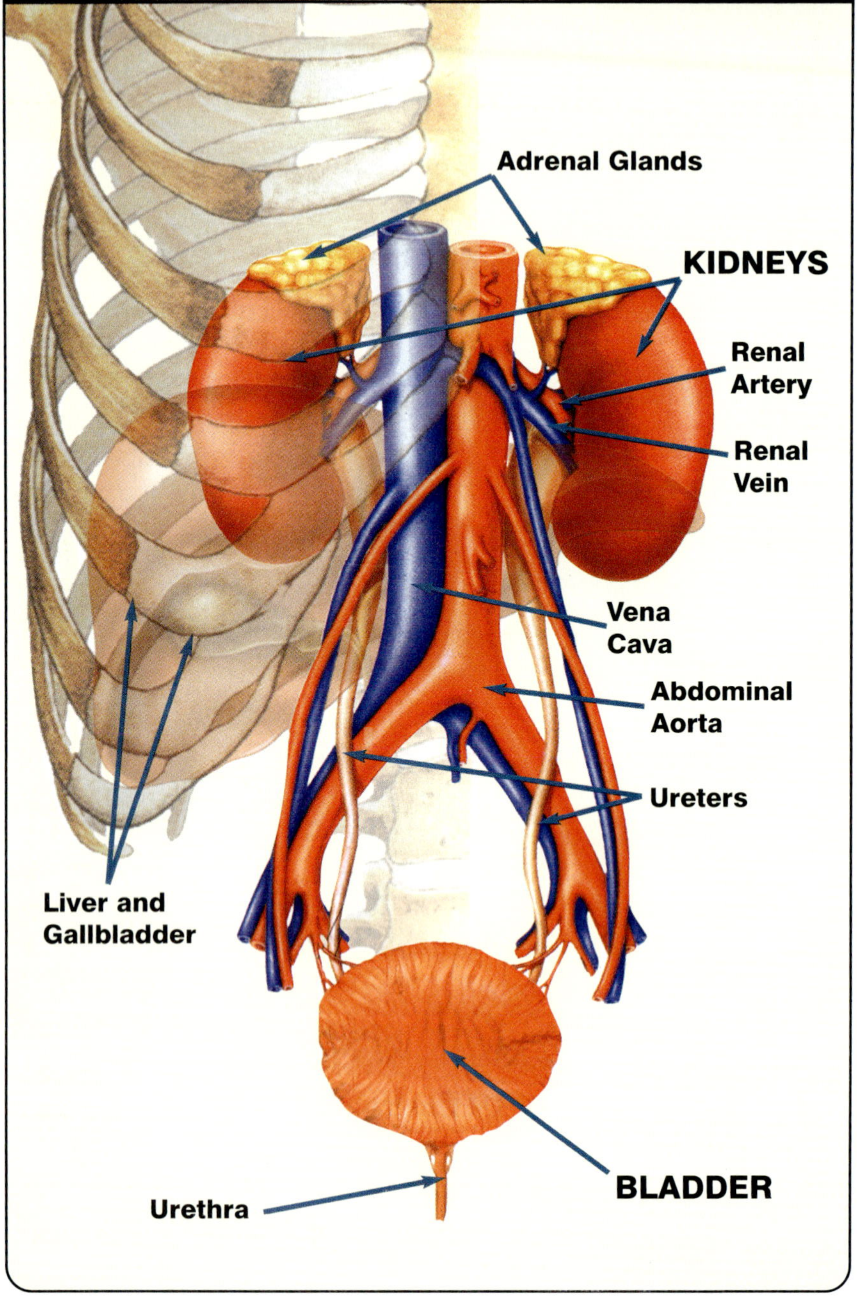

CHAPTER TWO

Anatomy and Physiology of the KIDNEYS AND BLADDER

At Last, a basic understanding of your Kidneys, Bladder and Urinary System that your medical doctor wouldn't tell you. And even if medical doctors did talk to their patients and explain things, you would need a dictionary in Greek, Latin, late Latin, French, ancient Anglo-Saxon, Old English, & numerous other languages and scientific terminology to decipher all their secret code words.

I have broken down all of their ten dollar words so you can understand the basics of what your Kidneys and Urinary Bladder look like, where they are, what they do and how they do it, at least as far as we know.

So don't be scared, take a deep breath, and in ten minutes you'll know all you'll need to know about peeing, and then some!

Very simply put, **the Urinary System is comprised of two Kidneys, one Bladder and a series of tubes.** The Kidneys look similar to Kidney beans in shape and also have a similar purple-brown color. They each weigh about 5 ounces and are about the same size as the palm of your hand, not including your fingers or thumb. You have one on each side of your spine. The top of each Kidney is about at the 12th Thoracic vertebra and the bottom being about at the 3rd Lumbar vertebra (from your mid to lower back). They are almost completely covered by your lowest back ribs.

The inner side (spinal side) of each Kidney has an indentation (the smaller curve of the Kidney shape) which is called the **hilus** or **hilum.** This is where all the tubes that take blood in and out, and urine out of your Kidneys connect and go into the Kidney, these being the **renal**

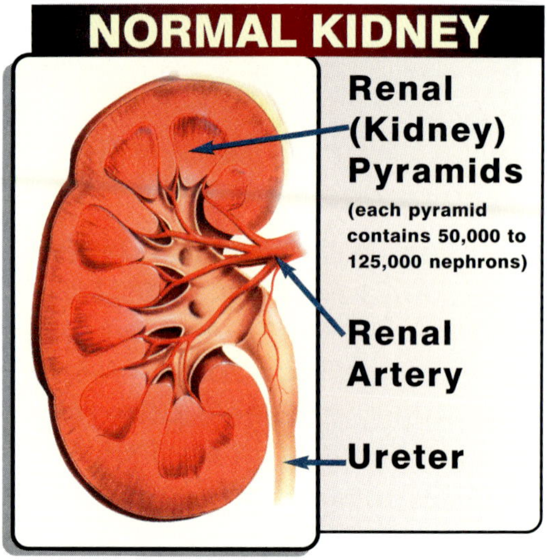

(*renalis* is Latin for Kidney) **artery**, the **renal vein** and the **ureter**. **The *Renal Artery* brings blood to the Kidney to be filtered and cleaned. The *Renal Vein* returns clean blood to your body and the waste liquid, urine, leaves the Kidney via the Ureter. Both the Ureters from each Kidney connect to the Bladder.** As with all metabolic processes of the human body, this process of blood filtering and urine formation is also very intricate, detailed, complex, and similar to when I talked about the Liver ***(see the companion book in this series, "Healing Liver and Gallbladder Disease Naturally")***. In other words, beyond mankind's comprehension. Knowing that, I will simplify this process so you have a basic understanding of what the Kidneys do and how they do it.

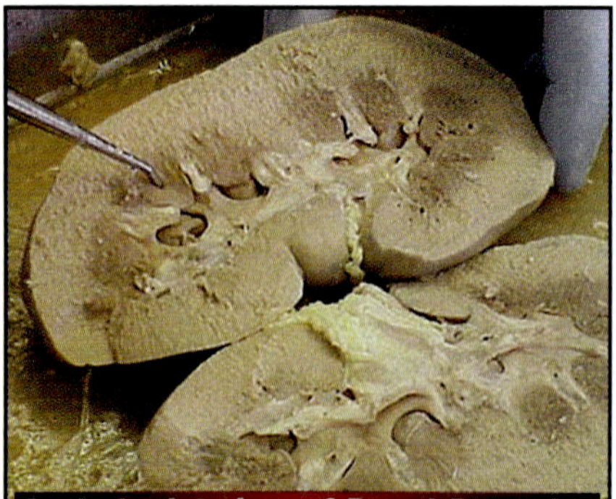
Pathologist view of Renal Pyramids

Each Kidney is divided into between 8 and 18 wedge- shaped chambers called **renal pyramids**. Each of these pyramids contains the many parts of the Kidney required to filter the blood. The outside of each **renal pyramid** is called the **renal cortex** (cortex is Latin for ***rind*** or ***outer edge***), and the inside closest to the **hilus** or smaller curve of the Kidney is called the **renal medulla** (medulla is Latin for ***inner*** or ***center***).

The **renal artery** branches off inside the Kidney to form numerous smaller arteries which enter the outer portion of the Kidney, the **renal cortex**. A very small renal artery branch eventually enters one of the many **Nephrons** (now that you know the Latin for Kidney, ***renalis*** hence renal**,** ***nephros*** is Greek for Kidney).

The Nephrons are the individual small filtering units in your Kidney and it is believed that each Kidney contains approximately one million of these Nephrons.

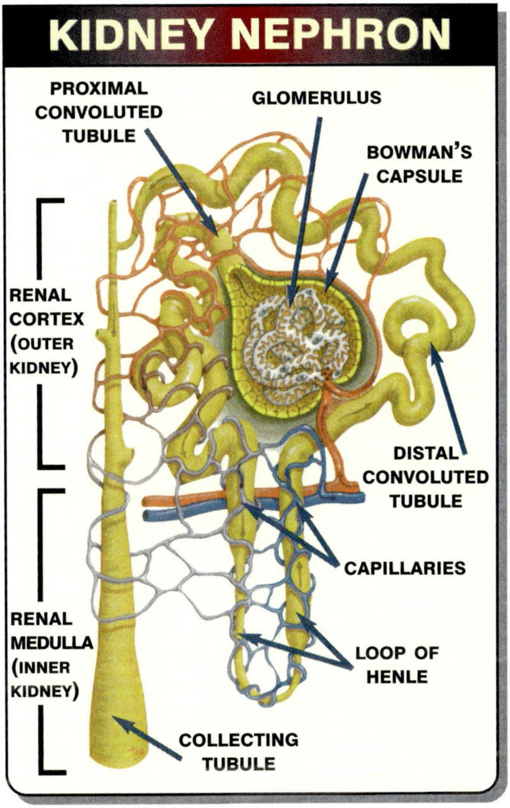

Inside each **Nephron** is a **renal corpuscle** and a **renal tubule.** The **renal corpuscle** is made up of a capillary network called a **glomerulus** enclosed in a **Bowman's capsule.** The **renal tubule** extends from the **Bowman's capsule** via the **proximal convoluted tubule**, the **loop of Henle,** the **distal convoluted tubule** and the **collecting tubule** all of which are surrounded and wrapped by **peritubular capillaries.**

NOTE: *capillaries, from the Latin* ***capillaris*** *meaning* ***hair-like,*** *are the smallest of the blood vessels/tubes, averaging 0.008mm in diameter which connect the very ends of the smallest arteries (arterioles) to the beginnings of the smallest veins (venules).*

Eventually the filtered blood waste (urine) enters into **collecting tubules** and then eventually the **papillary ducts** which are in the **renal medulla** or the inner or center portion of the Kidney. These **papillary ducts** eventually empty into the **ureter** through which the urine leaves the Kidney.

I know that for those of you who just want to do my Kidney/Bladder Flush Drink and Herbal Tonics this is not only anatomical overload but downright unappetizing, but hang in there with me for a few more minutes and it will begin to make some sense.

It is the Kidneys' job to filter blood plasma, return good blood to the body and create urine to carry waste out of the body. Your blood plasma is the liquid that your blood cells (including your red blood cells) swim around in.

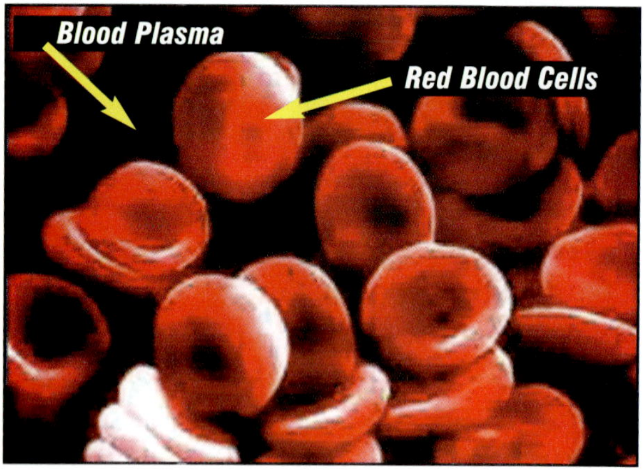

While many know that most cars have water-cooled engines, the human Kidney is a water run waste removal system. Much of the water that you consume is necessary to clean the blood and flush waste material out of the body via the Kidneys. The Kidneys also regulate the water, electrolyte and acid/alkaline balance of the blood and, indirectly, all body fluids.

HOW IT ALL WORKS

Blood enters your Kidneys in the inner indented section **(hilus)** closest to the spine via the **renal artery.** Inside of your Kidney this artery divides down into many other smaller arteries that enter one of the pyramid shaped separate kidney chambers **(renal pyramid),** and branch down into even smaller arteries in the **renal cortex**. One of these small arteries enters a very small microscopic sac **(nephron),** which is an individual filtering unit. As blood passes inside the **nephron** into the **renal corpuscle,** through the **glomerulus** and **Bowman's capsule,** water and dissolved substances and small bits are filtered out of the blood but big things like blood cells and large proteins are retained in the **capillaries** and blood. As the water and dissolved substances that were filtered out of the blood, which is now called **glomerular filtrate** (we could call this pre-pee) passes through the **renal tubules**, the **proximal convoluted tubule**, the **loop of Henle,** the **distal convoluted tubule** and the **collecting tubule,** it moves into the other area of the Kidney called the **renal medulla.** Here the urine goes into the **papillary ducts** and eventually leaves the Kidneys through the **ureter.**

Useful materials such as water, glucose, amino acids, vitamins and minerals are reabsorbed into the blood via the small **capillaries**. This reabsorbing is monitored and limited by your body. The reabsorbing of nutrients is stopped if you have too much of a nutrient already and the reabsorbing of water is regulated by hormones.

The Kidneys are the organ mainly responsible for not only the filtering of the blood, but they also regulate the physical properties and composition of the blood by monitoring the acid-alkaline balance. What is left in the remaining liquid that is now called urine is about 95% water and 5% dissolved substances. The dissolved substances are minerals, especially sodium, nitrogenous waste products like urea, uric acid, creatine, creatinine, ammonia, chlorides, calcium, magnesium, phosphorous and many other substances like blood, pus, bacteria, parasites, all depending on the disease or health level of the person.

The urine leaves each Kidney via the **ureter** and both right and left Kidney ureters connect to the Bladder separately, on the corresponding side. The Bladder is a general term from the Anglo-Saxon ***blaedre*** meaning a sac or receptacle for a secretion, like the **gallbladder**. The **urinary bladder** then, of course, is the muscular receptacle for urine, and without it your urine would just constantly run out of your body. The Bladder is in the lower front of your pelvic cavity. In women it is in front of the vagina and in men in front of the rectum.

The Bladder has a normal storage capacity of about a quart or more. When the Bladder fills, it stretches, which initiates nerve impulses to the spinal cord. When you want to urinate, returning motor nerve impulses simultaneously cause contraction of the bladder and relaxation of the bladder sphincter muscle. This process can be stopped temporarily by the voluntary contraction of the external urethral sphincter muscle.

At the very bottom of the Bladder is the **urethra**, a tube that the urine passes through to leave the body. On the man this tube passes through the center of the prostate gland and out through the center of the penis and out the end. It is also used for the passage of semen. This is why when a man has a swollen prostate due to sexual function or disease, it squeezes off the urethra making voiding urine very difficult. In a woman, the urethra leaves the bladder and the orifice where the urine is voided is in the vestibule between the vagina and the clitoris.

OK, enough is enough. Knowing a few of the details can not only help you understand your illness if you have Kidney Disease, but also will help you to understand when I explain my Kidney and Bladder Cleansing, Detoxification and Healing Programs.

DIAGNOSIS OF DISEASE OF THE URINARY SYSTEM

THE "AMOUNT" OF URINE

Normally a person should urinate about 4 to 6 times a day. This amount can vary greatly depending on the amount of liquids you consume, how much you weigh, how much you are exercising, breathing, sweating, etc. The average person eliminates between 1 and 2 quarts of urine a day. Any change in the amount of urine excreted can be a sign that something is wrong with the Urinary System.

THE "LOOK AND SMELL" OF THE URINE

Since recorded history, people have noticed that another sign of Urinary System disease is a change in color, transparency and smell of the urine, so examining urine was something all doctors did thousands of years before modern medicine. I have studied with many traditional doctors that would examine urine with just their eyes and nose and diagnose many diseases and metabolic imbalances better than many modern urologists with their high tech laboratories. Even modern medical texts contain pages of descriptions of urine colors and smells to help doctors diagnose urinary illness. Just a few of the colors in medical text are Blue, Black, Bile-colored, Colorless, Lime Green, Milky, Orange-Red, Pale, Red, Reddish, and the odors listed are endless, from Fishy and New-Mown Hay to Over Ripe Apples.

So again, any changes in urine quantity, color, transparency, odor, specific gravity, dilution ability and acidity can be a warning sign that your body is out of balance and your Kidneys are unhappy, and starting to be damaged.

If you are interested in further study of disease diagnosis from changes in the urine read ***"Ancient Healing Wisdom Blows Away Modern Technology"*** *on page 38 or consult your local medical university bookstore.*

ALL diseases and imbalances that cause the destruction of the Kidneys can be totally REVERSED.

I repeat, ALL of these diseases and imbalances that cause the destruction of the Kidneys can be totally REVERSED.

I have always said:

"GETTING WELL IS SIMPLE –
STOP doing what is making you sick.
START to do what will heal your body."

CHAPTER THREE

KIDNEY and BLADDER DISEASE

DISEASES THAT CAUSE URINARY SYSTEM BREAKDOWN & ILLNESS

TOXEMIA

Most damage to the Kidneys and their ability to filter and clean your blood is caused by Toxemia, excessively dirty blood, the result of a degenerative lifestyle.

If your blood has too much toxic waste in it, it is very hard on your Kidneys. This can be caused by being constipated and having pounds of old fecal matter in your bowel and reabsorbing the poisons back into your blood: ***auto-intoxication***. Your food program may also be too high in junk food that is laden with toxic and poisonous chemicals from preservatives to insecticides. With a high level of poisons and toxins in your bloodstream, from your retained waste and your food program, your Kidneys don't stand a chance and can't handle the filtering job. <u>They are just plain overloaded.</u> It is like expecting your oil filter in your car to do its job, but you haven't changed your oil in 100,000 miles and the oil is filled with impurities. Your oil filter (Kidney) is just going to fail, quit, and your oil (blood) is just going to stay dirty until your engine (body) fails.

All of this toxic waste buildup in your Kidneys is a leading cause of Kidney and Bladder Cancer.

If this is you, make sure that along with my ***5-Day Cleansing and Detoxification Program,*** *using the* ***Kidney/Bladder Flush*** *and my* ***Kidney/Bladder Formula*** *(Chapters Four & Five), you also do my* ***Bowel Detoxification Program*** *(see* ***"Healing Colon Disease Naturally"****) and start a Healthy Food Program.*

HYPER-CHOLESTEROLEMIA AND HYPERTENSION

Your Liver and Gallbladder may be congested, overloaded and plugged because your food program is too high in Animal Foods. This causes hyper-cholesterolemia (high cholesterol levels) which in turn causes hypertension (high blood pressure). High blood pressure causes almost half of all Kidney Disease.

Your Kidneys have a much harder time filtering out thick fatty blood than filtering out thinner blood. This is just basic physics. Try pouring water through a coffee filter. It will run through the filter very fast. Now try pouring in and filtering ice cream or cheese. Not very easy is it, saturated fat from animal foods makes your blood very thick, increasing your cholesterol level and therefore making it very difficult for your Kidneys to filter your blood. In fact, it will clog the tiny filtering capillaries and nephrons in your Kidneys, rendering them incapable of filtering anything.

This fatty blood is also much harder for your heart to pump around your body so your heart has to increase its pumping force(your blood pressure).Again this is basic physics. If you are pumping water through a pipe 100 feet long and now you want to pump cheese instead, it will take more pressure to pump a thicker mass. This causes high blood pressure and this higher pressure ruptures and hemorrhages the very tiny capillaries and microscopic parts of your Kidney's blood filtering system, scarring them and eventually killing them.

*If this is you, make sure that along with my **5-Day Cleansing and Detoxification Program,** using the **Kidney/Bladder Flush Drink** and **Kidney/Bladder Formula,** you also do my Liver and Gallbladder Cleansing (see **Healing Liver and Gallbladder Disease Naturally**) and begin a Healthy Vegetarian Food Program.*

DIABETES

High Blood Sugar, ***Diabetes,*** causes almost the other half of Kidney Disease that High Blood Pressure doesn't. There are many known ways in which high blood sugar hurts the Kidneys and many additional theories. Again, the micro-filtration systems of the Kidneys are very fragile to blood viscosity, pressure, toxic waste and severe blood imbalances like Diabetes. Diabetics have excessive urination, hence the name Diabetes, ***(from the Greek meaning passing through).*** These comprise just some of the reasons being a Diabetic can cause the rupture, breakdown and eventual scarring and lesions on the small delicate Kidney filtering micro parts and render them at first, incapacitated, and eventually incompetent and dead.

In my clinic I treated hundreds of Diabetics, all of whom if they were willing to go far enough, got their Diabetes under control and off of any insulin with a Healthy Food Program, Exercise and routine Cleansing and Detoxification Programs.

DEATH ROW DIALYSIS

Kidney Dialysis is really a death sentence, like a ticking time bomb. After 5 years on dialysis only about 1/4 of the people are left alive. After 10 years, less than 8 percent are still living. ***On dialysis you actually die sooner than the average person rotting to death with malignant cancer.*** Whether you know it or not your doctor is just waiting for someone else to die so they can cut a Kidney out and sew it into you. On average, this cadaver kidney and you will be dead in 9 years.

NORMAL KIDNEY

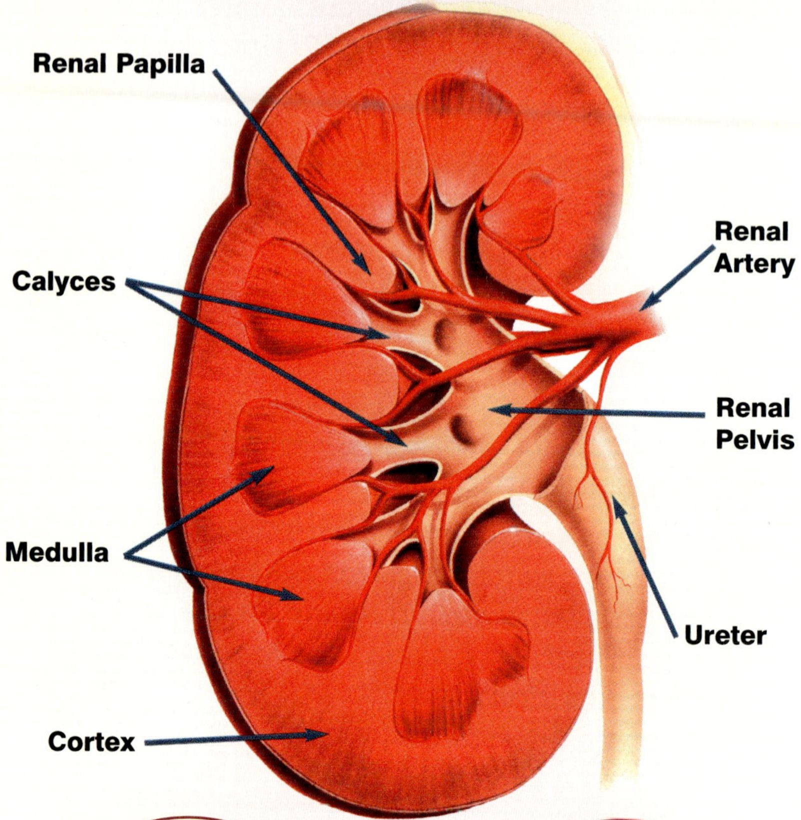

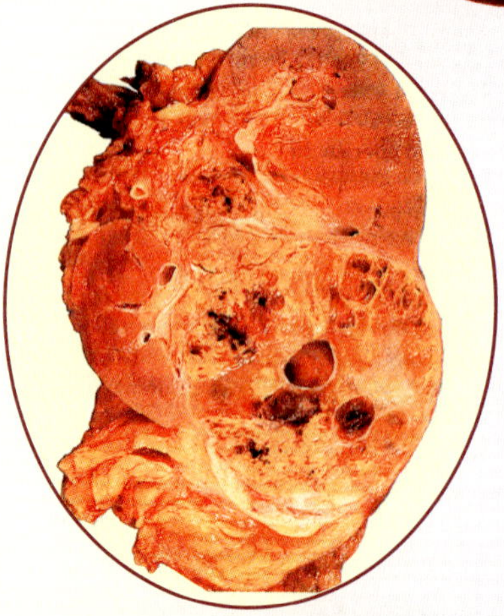

KIDNEY CANCER

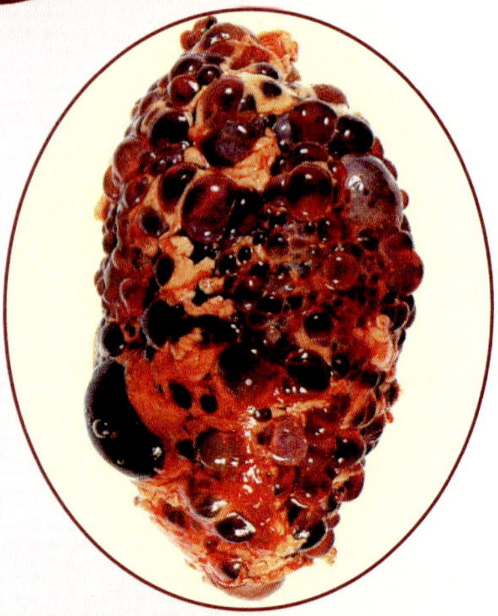

POLYCYSTIC KIDNEY

DISEASES of the KIDNEYS

THE BOTTOM LINE ON ANY KIDNEY, BLADDER OR URINARY SYSTEM DISEASE

I have seen a lot of strange things in my life, especially in my clinic, but I've never seen a Kidney walk into my office, lie down on my examination table and say, ***"Doc, I don't feel so good."***

Early in my practice I realized that there is a whole person in my office and that **the real problem is probably NOT where the pain is, and true healing is getting to the cause of disease.**

Medical doctors have a bad habit of looking at where the pain is or where the final breakdown occurs. So with Kidney disease, the medical doctor reacts by looking at the Kidneys, seeing that they are failing, inflamed or falling apart and then suggests Kidney medications, dialysis and eventually Kidney transplantation. This is as stupid as if you put cola, coffee or cow's milk in the gas tank of your car and then blamed the engine when it quits running. Sure the engine doesn't work, and may be damaged, but the cause of the problem is **NOT** the engine. The engine can run again just by flushing and cleaning it out and putting some proper fuel in the tank. Any greasemonkey kid knows this. Maybe we should make all medical doctors take a year of basic auto repair before they start their pre-med curriculum.

Even if the medical doctor realizes that your Kidneys are self-destructing because of your high blood pressure or fatty blood, most doctors think this is just the normal disease process of the American lifestyle and that you are incapable of any modification – especially the taking on of some

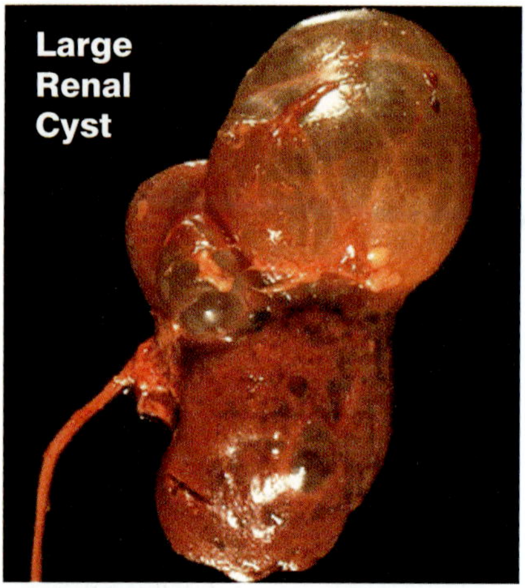

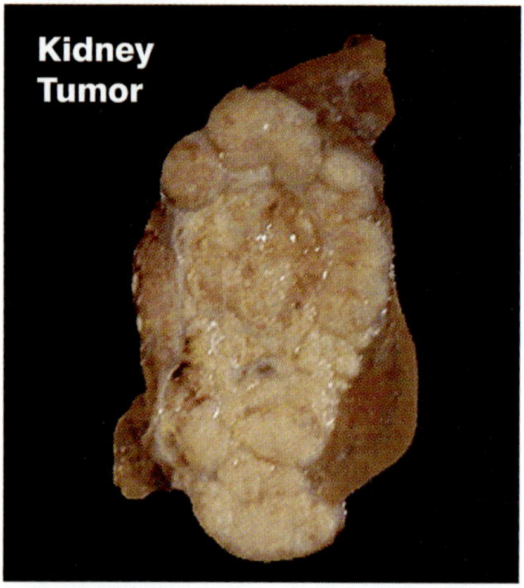

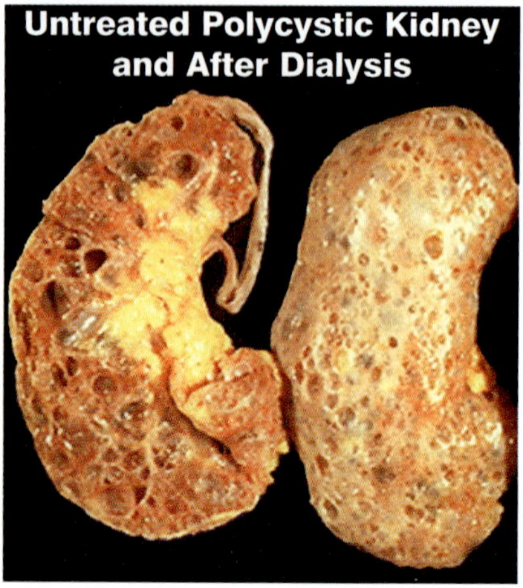

"A Picture is Worth 1,000 Words"

radical, extremist health program, like eating less meat, drinking a little juice and walking. Consequently medical doctors rarely suggest any changes in your lifestyle. They try to HEAL your Kidneys or any failing organ, **without your help!** This only buys time, but never heals.

The only reason your Kidneys are failing is because the blood they are trying to filter is more like a toxic sludge. If you clean up your lifestyle, your food program, flush out your elimination organs *(especially your Bowel, your Liver and Gallbladder and of course your Kidneys)* your Kidneys and your body will heal itself.

KIDNEY STONES

"When I was a kid I remember hearing my dad screaming in pain in the toilet, and then coming out in about 15 minutes, totally soaked in sweat. I later discovered that he had passed a Kidney Stone. For those of you that have never passed a stone, you don't want to know the pain and torture of it all. Although I have never personally passed one, I had many patients that had, some right in the bathroom of my clinic. Most described it as a pain so severe that it took their breath away, Some dropped right to the floor crying and screaming. There is no running away from it and it feels like you are peeing a combination of sharp broken glass and boiling acid. From the amount of blood in some of my patients' urine, it looked like they were bleeding to death. Not a pleasant experience at all."

Because the Kidneys try to filter acids and minerals out of your blood, but get over loaded as I stated earlier, you can get a buildup of mineral gravel, stones, acid crystals and mineral plaque inside your Kidneys. This sediment can build up over years and turn into rocks, but also literally turn your Kidneys into petrified rock. It can take over your entire Kidney structure and eventually become fossilized. ***(See the picture below.)***

The vast majority of all Kidney stones is made up of Calcium. Isn't this interesting, while we all seem to be trying to get more Calcium into our diets?

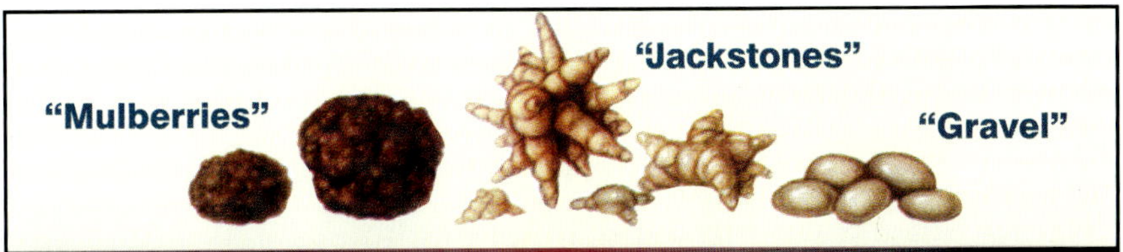

Different Kidney Stones

KIDNEY STONES

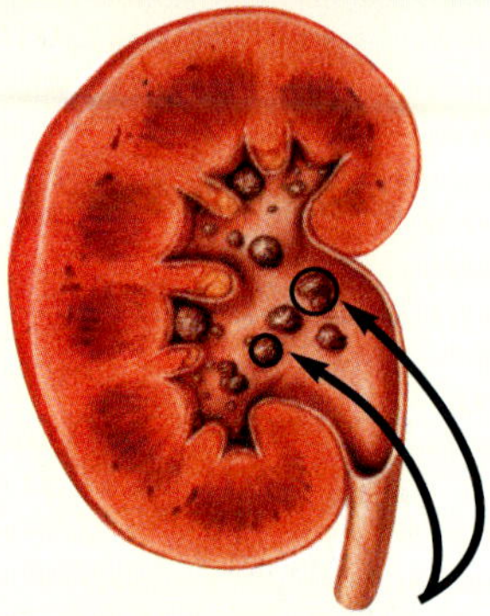

70% OF ALL STONES ARE CALCIUM STONES

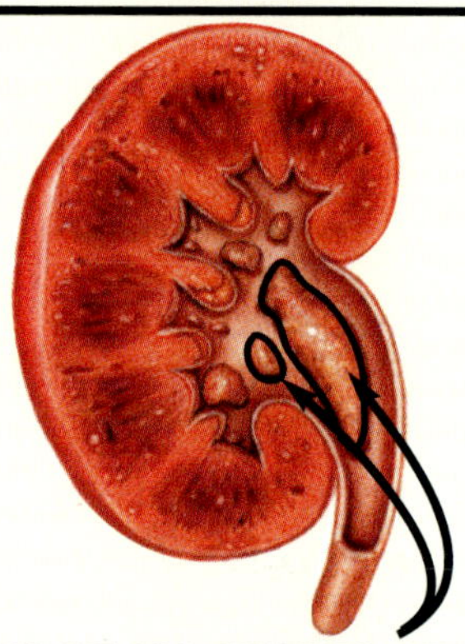

15% OF ALL STONES ARE URIC ACID STONES

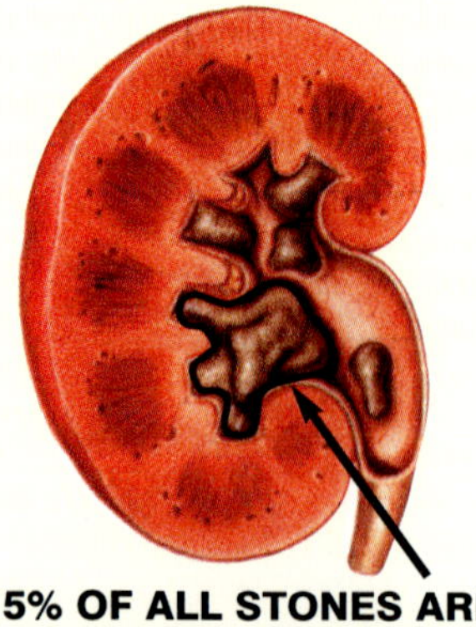

15% OF ALL STONES ARE MAGNESIUMAMMONIUM PHOSPHATE STONES

In many people's attempts to get more calcium into their bodies, ironically, they actually lose more instead. This often happens when women, worried about osteoporosis, start drinking more milk and eating more dairy products.

Animal food is very high in calcium, but also very high in protein. When you consume it, as part of the digestive process of any high protein food, you often end up peeing out more calcium as your body attempts to utilize all this protein. All this calcium pouring out of your blood and flooding through your Kidneys actually overloads your Kidneys with Calcium. And remember, over 70% of all Kidney stones are Calcium Rocks!

So what you want to do is not only get more calcium into your mouth, but also to get calcium that will stay in your blood and eventually get into your bones – not get urinated away. This is why Low Protein but High Calcium foods are much better choices and we can retain the calcium in our blood.

Carrots, citrus and greens are much better choices than high protein milk and dairy products. Ounce for ounce, organic carrot juice made at home right in your own juicer has as much if not more calcium than cow's milk, and you don't pee all the calcium into the toilet. Plus it tastes better. If you are not used to the taste of carrot juice, then mix it with a little apple, or a lot of apple at first until you get used to it. This is also a great way to get the kids drinking carrot juice: 90% fresh organic apple and 10% fresh organic carrot; any kid will love that.

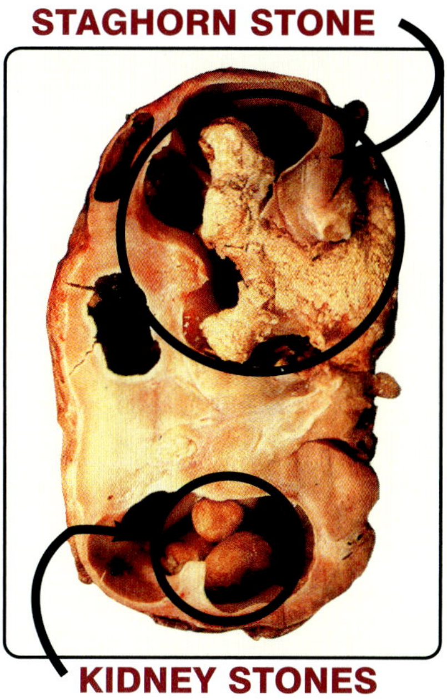

NOTE: *This same calcium plaque that causes Kidney stones also builds up in coronary arteries and cerebral arteries along with cholesterol, causing heart attacks and strokes, again caused by a high animal food diet.*

The latest fad high protein diets, like the Atkin's and the Zone, can take people's weight off, but it can also turn your Kidneys to stone. Most medical books suggest the first place to look when a patient has Kidney stones is the diet and if they are on a high protein diet, get them off it immediately. (Recently the tabloids have been full of reports about Hollywood stars having to be hospitalized for hurting their Kidneys with these high-protein weight loss diets.)

Other stones are formed from Uric Acid and actually form Uric Acid Crystals in the Kidneys. Again, this buildup is often caused by a bad diet, high in animal foods which contain tons of uric acid along with processed foods, junk foods, etc.

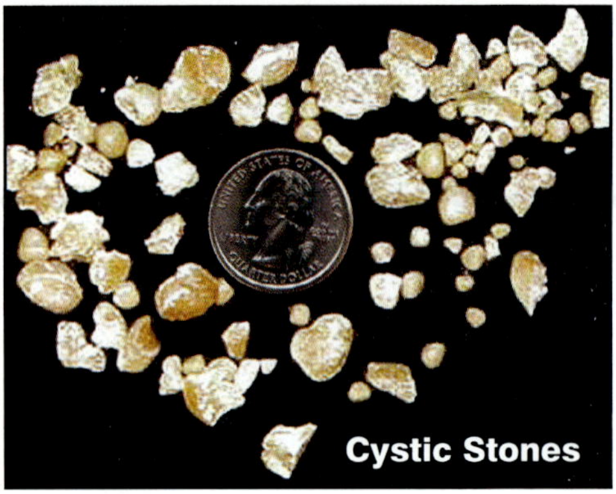

Most medical texts state that Alkalinization of the urine through diet can dissolve Uric Acid crystals and stones. In my clinic I would use both the Alkalinization of the urine through a raw food and juice program **(Dr. Schulze's 5-Day Cleansing and Detoxification Program)** and foods and herbs that dissolve urinary stones and gravel (**Dr. Schulze's Kidney and Bladder Herbal Formula and Tea** to dissolve all types of stones, Uric Acid, Calcium; **EVERY TYPE OF STONE!)**

Remember, the Alkalinization of the urine and blood has nothing to do with the ph (acid or alkaline) level of a particular food, but how the food reacts to your body's metabolism. In other words, acidic foods with a low ph like citrus and apple cider vinegar actually have a very strong alkalizing effect on your urine and blood. Generally, foods

IF YOU DON'T WANT ROCKS and GRAVEL IN YOUR KIDNEYS, STOP EATING ROCKS and GRAVEL.

Since Calcium and Uric Acid is what most Kidney Stones are made of, then just by stopping eating animal foods you can halt the formation of stones. Refraining from eating stones, gravel and dirt is also very helpful.

Since most mineral supplements are made from rocks, gravel, stones, pulverized oyster shells, old animal bones and even metal, eliminating this junk mineral supplementation can also prevent the formation of Kidney Stones. I would put all of my patients that either had Kidney Stones or a family history of them on my **SuperFood.** The minerals in **SuperFood** will give you a nutrient blast, but will not contribute to the formation of stones. In fact, **SuperFood** will alkalinize your blood which will actually help you to dissolve stones.

that have an alkalizing effect on your body fluids are Fruits, Vegetables, Sprouts, Raw Foods and Juices. Foods that have an acidifying effect are animal foods, processed foods, sugar, junk food; you know, the bad stuff.

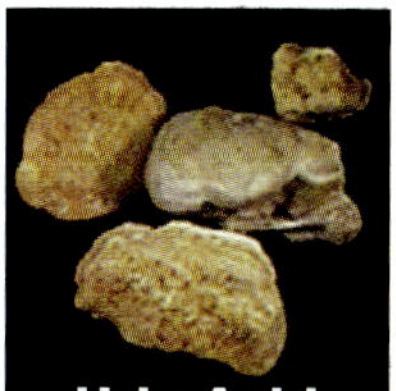
Uric Acid Stones

So getting on a good raw food and juice program can dissolve stones, rocks, crystals and any kind of sediment in your Kidneys.

Uric Acid Crystals in the Kidneys are easy to dissolve quickly. Small calcium gravel and plaque is easier and faster to dissolve than one large stone. Regardless of the size of your crystal and rock collection, if you have or even suspect any type of sediment, gravel or stone in your Kidneys or Bladder, or have been diagnosed by a doctor as having them, it is time to get to work.

As a minimum, do my **5-Day Cleansing and Detoxification Program** on pages 10 and 11 that includes the Kidney/Bladder Flush Drink and all of the **Kidney/ Bladder Herbal Formulae.**

APPLES, THE DISSOLVER OF CALCIUM AND URIC ACID STONES: A DR. SCHULZE DEMONSTRATION

Fill a canning jar about three quarters of the way up with apple cider vinegar (acetic acid) or use white vinegar which is clearer and makes it easier to see. (I never advise consuming white vinegar – only for this experiment). Place a chicken egg into the solution. (I know this is gross and you may be a vegan so borrow an egg from a neighbor; a picture can be worth a thousand words.) Within a few days the vinegar will dissolve all of the eggshell which is made of calcium, but it will not harm or dissolve the thin membrane that holds the egg together. In this same way, phytochemicals in Raw Apple Juice and Apple Cider Vinegar can dissolve calcium stones in your Kidneys, but never harm nor irritate the delicate membranes.

If the problem still persists I suggest doing my 5-Day Cleansing and Detoxification Routine for an additional week. You can also do my Stone Dissolving Routine ***(on this page)*** that I used in my clinic to dissolve literally thousands of Kidney stones.

DISEASES of the BLADDER

BLADDER INFECTIONS: *THE STATISTICS*

One of the most common types of all infections in men and women are Bladder Infections. They are sometimes referred to as cystitis (kystis is the Greek for Bladder and itis for inflammation) Women are 50 times more likely to get bladder infections than men. 95% of bladder infections are caused by bacteria entering the opening of the urethra that literally travel up the urethral opening into the bladder. About 80% of these bacterial infections are caused by the gram-negative Escherichia coli bacteria (E. coli) and the rest usually by other well known bacteria.

In my clinic I saw two major reasons for Bladder infections, especially in women, and both were based on sexual activity. Most common was when one of my single female patients had not been sexually active for a time and then met Mr. Right and had a weekend fling in Santa Barbara where they made love just about all weekend long. During sexual intercourse lots of generally benign bacteria that are very common to the male and female body, like E. coli, are spread around the vaginal and urethral openings. Just urinating will flush these bacteria out of the urethra and prevent a bacterial infection. But sometimes couples fall asleep after intercourse and sleep all night, maybe wake up and do it again, but in either case this gives the bacteria time to work its way up into the bladder. No

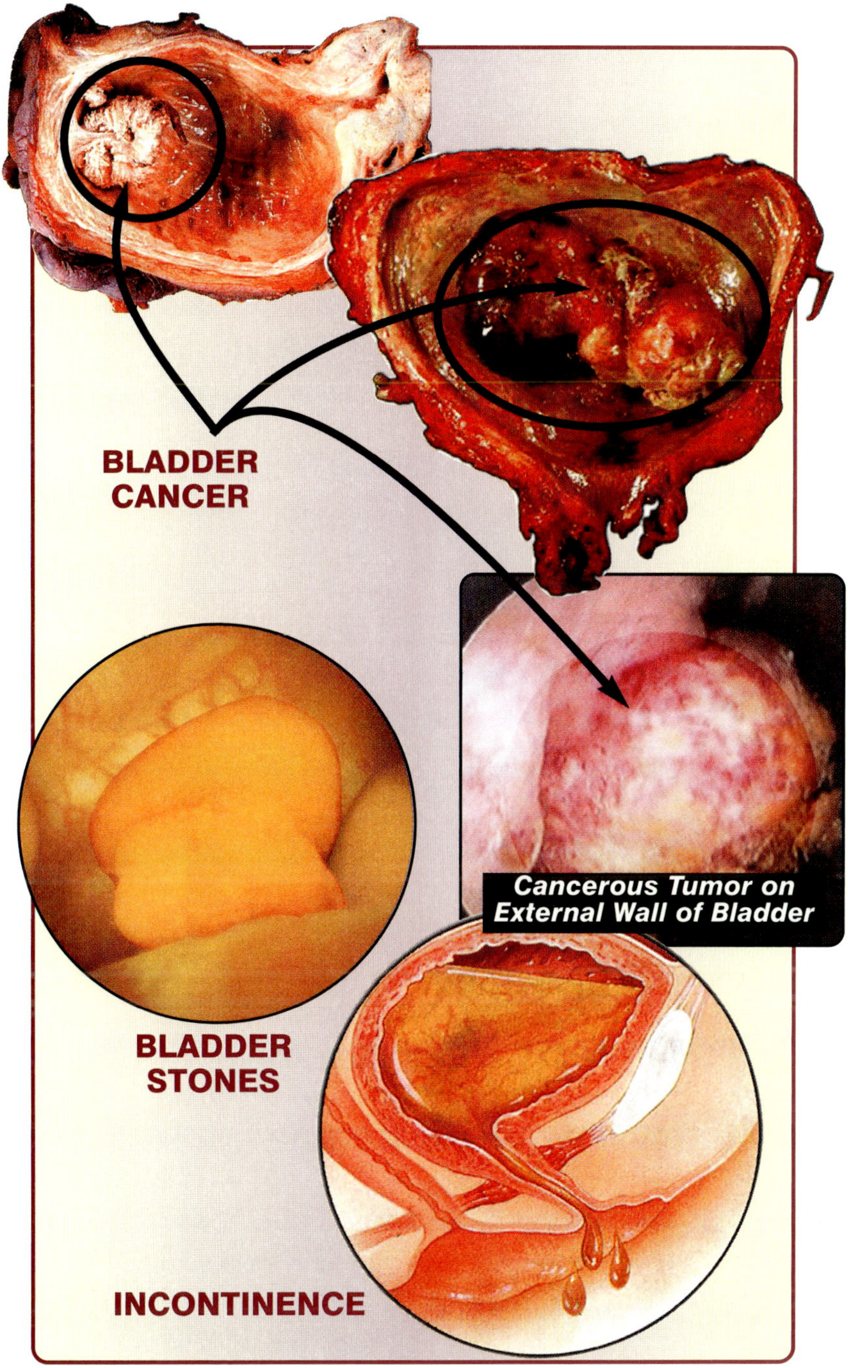
BLADDER CANCER
Cancerous Tumor on External Wall of Bladder
BLADDER STONES
INCONTINENCE

matter how un-romantic this sounds, GET UP AND PEE soon after intercourse. This will reduce your chances of getting a bladder infection to almost nothing.

The other most common cause of bladder infections is antibiotics, spermicides (used for diaphrams and on condoms) or any other medication that is proven to imbalance your vaginal bacterial flora and permit the overgrowth of E. coli bacteria.

In any case, men, women, sexually active or celibate, cystitis or bladder infections and even infections of the urethra or ureter are treated exactly the same as kidney infections by following my Kidney/Bladder Flush Drink and the 5-Day Kidney/Bladder Cleansing and Detoxification Program in Chapters Four and Five.

ANCIENT HEALING WISDOM *BLOWS AWAY* MODERN TECHNOLOGY

Many years ago while working in a clinic in Asia, I was told of a rural doctor that had an almost perfect success rate at diagnosing Urinary Tract diseases and many other illnesses from studying his patient s urine. I traveled to visit his clinic which to my surprise was not much more than a mud hut. He would ask the patient to urinate into a cup. After the patient gave him a urine sample he would walk out the back door of the hut, come back through the door in a few minutes and have his diagnosis, which according to what I observed was incredibly accurate.

When I asked him if I could observe his laboratory tests and evaluations he invited me through the back door of his hut to a small table and chair out back. The first thing he would do was look at the urine in the clear glass with the sun behind it and study the color. Next he would take a long, deep sniff, similar to a wine taster deeply inhaling a fine chardonnay, and would then often mumble something. He would then proceed to pour some of the patient s urine on an ant hill and then take the leftover to the table where he first divided it into two bowls then proceeded to drop various herb powders and grains into the urine. In a few minutes he went back and checked the ant hill and then the urine on the table in the bowls and then without hesitation walked back into the hut and gave his incredibly accurate diagnosis. After a few days I figured some of his genius out.

First he checked the color and transparency of the urine which can tell you everything from Liver disease and Kidney inflammation to poisoning. He then smelled the urine which can give you a hundred more clues. The human eyes and nose are still much more sensitive than any laboratory equipment ever developed, although many doctors don t like to admit it. The rate at which his ants were attracted or repelled by the urine told him many things, but definitely the amount of sugar in the urine. Diabetes is the #1 cause of Kidney disease so he needed to rule that out. Dropping herb powders in the bowls of urine samples told him many things from specific gravity to dilution ability which are both tests for Kidney and Pancreatic disease. He also could tell the acidity of the urine by which certain herbal flowers changed color which can tell you everything from infections to low grade fevers. All I can say is a few days with this man taught me more than a year in a hospital lab, especially in using my favorite diagnostic protocols of ***simplicity and common sense.***

"First of all, no one but God really understands the kidneys, the bladder, and the urinary tract. All the systems of the human body are way too complex for us to even begin to understand.

But on a basic level I can get you to understand them enough to figure out and see what's going on, to make a good common sense decision, and once you use your common sense, you'll see that the real healing, the true healing...is all YOU healing YOUrself."

- Dr. Richard Schulze

CHAPTER FOUR

THE SOLUTION
Dr. Schulze's KIDNEY/BLADDER Flush Drink

The Kidney and Bladder Flush and my Kidney and Bladder Herbal formula have many healing benefits to your Urinary System.

First, just by consuming all the liquid you are literally flushing the Kidneys out. Just by urinating more you can remove infections and stones in the Kidneys and Bladder. This is very important, especially first thing in the morning since your Kidneys have been sleeping and near dormant all night long. In the morning you most likely have a higher bacteria count and higher level of sediment in your Kidneys than any other time.

The citrus juices in the Kidney Flush not only supply you with needed electrolytes, but will alkalize your blood which is proven to dissolve uric acid crystals and even Kidney stones. They also help to flush out mucous and are diuretic, making you urinate more.

This flush is based on a wonderful old drink by Stanley Burroughs called the Master Cleanser which was successful in helping thousands of people heal themselves of many different diseases.

The citrus juices contain citric acid but apple cider vinegar contains acetic acid and can be used as a replacement if you cannot get good quality fresh citrus fruit. The apple cider vinegar must be raw, organic and unfiltered like Bragg's or Spectrum. It will have the same action.

The Herbs in my Kidney and Bladder Formula and my Kidney and Bladder Herb Tea have 3 major actions: Diuretic, Disinfectant and Dissolving. Herbs such as Uva

Ursi Leaves, Juniper Berries, Corn Silk, Horsetail Herb, Parsley Leaf and Root, Carrot Tops, and others in the formula have been used for centuries as Diuretics ***(herbs that make you urinate more)***. Even today, most of these herbs are listed in medical and chemistry books for this action. Some of these herbs, like Juniper Berries and Uva Ursi Leaves, contain phytochemicals like volatile oils that are also powerfully disinfectant and destroy bacteria that lives in your Kidneys and Bladder and therefore are healing for Kidney and Bladder Infections. Herbs like Hydrangea root and Gravel Root are famous for their ability to dissolve Kidney stones. So the Kidney/Bladder Flush Drink makes you urinate more, disinfects the Kidneys and Bladder and dissolves and flushes out any sediment before it turns into rocks. And if you already have rocks, it starts breaking them down and dissolving them.

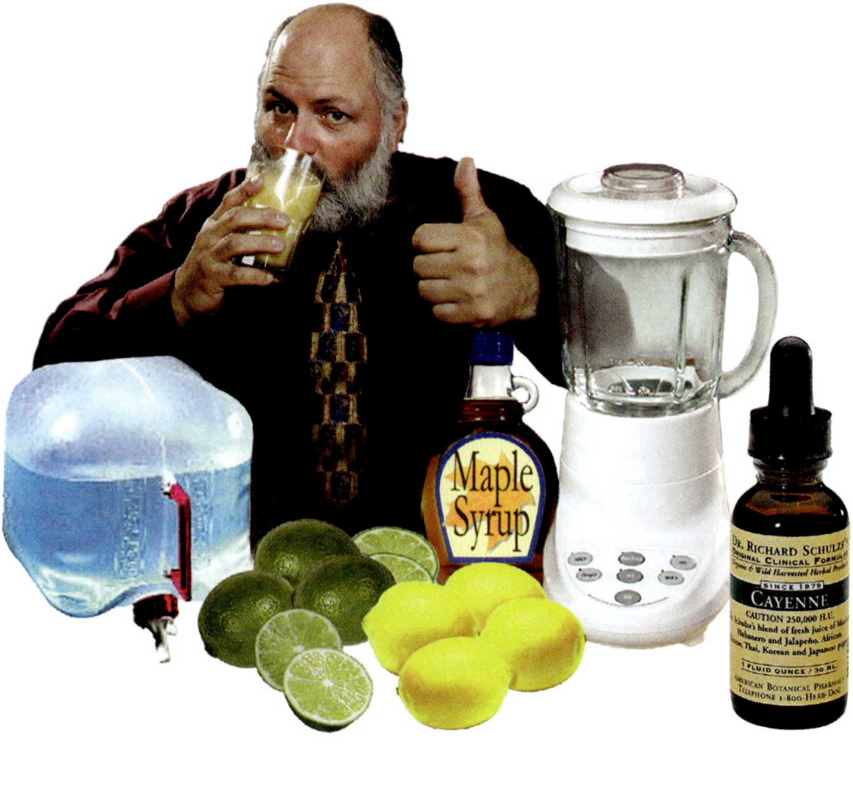

HOW TO MAKE DR. SCHULZE'S 2 MINUTE KIDNEY AND BLADDER FLUSH DRINK

PUT THESE INGREDIENTS IN A BLENDER:

1. **16 - 32 ounces of distilled or purified water.**
2. **Juice of 1 lemon and 1 lime.**
3. **A pinch of Dr. Schulze's CAYENNE POWDER or 5-20 drops of Dr. Schulze's *Famous* CAYENNE TINCTURE.**
4. ***Optional:* A small amount of maple syrup to taste.**
5. **Blend on high speed for 10-15 seconds.**
6. **CONSUME THIS DRINK.**

***NOTE:* It only takes me 60 seconds to make my KIDNEY FLUSH DRINK in the morning. Drink the flush down in 2-3 minutes. Don't sip it.**

AFTER DRINKING YOUR FLUSH

- **15-20 minutes after drinking your Kidney Flush, drink 2 cups of previously prepared KIDNEY/BLADDER HERB TEA** (see directions on page 52).
- **Put 2 droppersful of my KIDNEY/BLADDER FORMULA in each cup of tea (consume a total of 4 droppersful) or have the tonic separately in an ounce of water.**

CHAPTER FIVE

THE SOLUTION Dr. Schulze's 5-Day KIDNEY/BLADDER Cleansing and Detoxification Program

YES, I designed my **5-Day Cleansing and Detoxification Program** to be done during the week, at work or during your regular weekly routine. Look, nobody wants to do a cleanse or detox on the weekend, and usually if you are silly enough to plan it that way, the phone rings, friends or relatives call, and the next thing you've blown it. Weekend fun, friends, parties, eating is a big part of all of this. During the week you are all very busy at work. You can do this program at work and you will hardly even notice that you've done it, IT WILL FLY BY. You might even set an example for a few of your co-workers who would be nicer people with their kidneys and bladder cleaned out.

THE PROGRAM IS TWO DAYS OF A PURIFYING RAW FOOD PROGRAM AND THREE DAYS OF A JUICE FAST.

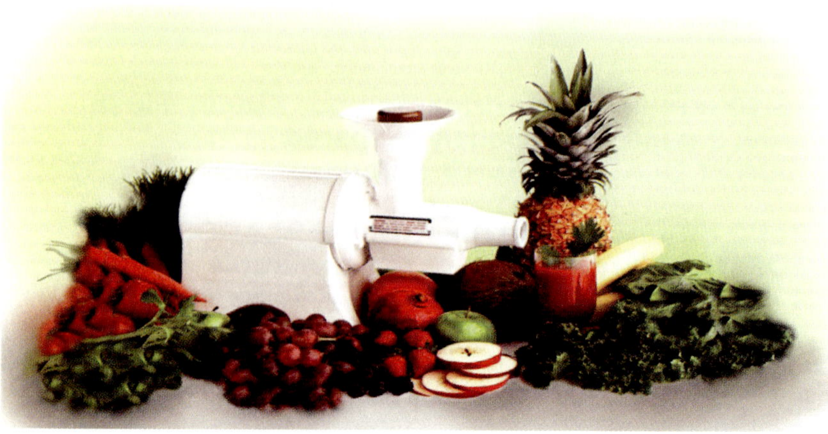

HOW TO DO MY 5-DAY KIDNEY/BLADDER CLEANSING and DETOXIFICATION PROGRAM

STEP 1: Upon arising drink 8 oz. of distilled or purified water.

STEP 2: Prepare and drink the **Kidney/Bladder Flush Drink**, and also prepare and drink the **Kidney/Bladder Tea** and **Kidney/ Bladder Formula** (see description on page 43).

STEP 3: Finally take 3 droppersful of my **D-Tox Formula**. This formula is my strongest tasting so you can put it in a little grape juice if you wish.

STEP 4: Repeat the same dosage of the **Kidney/Bladder Tea & Kidney/Bladder Formula** 2 more times during the day.

STEP 5: Repeat the same dosage of my **D-TOX Formula** 4 more times during the day.

STEP 6: One hour later drink your **SuperFood Morning Nutritional Drink.**

STEP 7: Continue with the **Food and Juice Program** as outlined next.

Remember to drink the **Kidney/Bladder Formula** and **Kidney/Bladder Tea** 2 more times during the day and take my **D-TOX Formula** 4 more times during the day.

FOOD & JUICE PROGRAM

Fresh fruit or vegetable juice is the best way to get your vitamins, minerals and other essential nutrients. They are also very important for cleansing and detoxification.

DAY #1 AND #5

Breakfast: If you're hungry before lunchtime you may have fruit, diluted fruit juice and fruit smoothies. Stop all fruit and fruit juice at least 1 hour before lunch. It is best while on this program not to mix fruits and vegetables.

Lunch: For lunch you can have fresh raw vegetable juices, raw vegetables alone or in salads, sprouts, potassium broth, and herb teas. You may use dressings for your salads and vegetables if you like, using olive oil, avocado, raw apple cider vinegar, lemon juice, garlic, onions, and any herbs and spices.

Afternoon snacks: Raw vegetables, raw vegetable salads, diluted vegetable juices, sprouts, potassium broth, and herb teas. All vegetable foods and juices must be stopped by 6pm.

Dinner: Diluted fruit juices, fruit, fruit smoothies, fruit salads and herb teas.

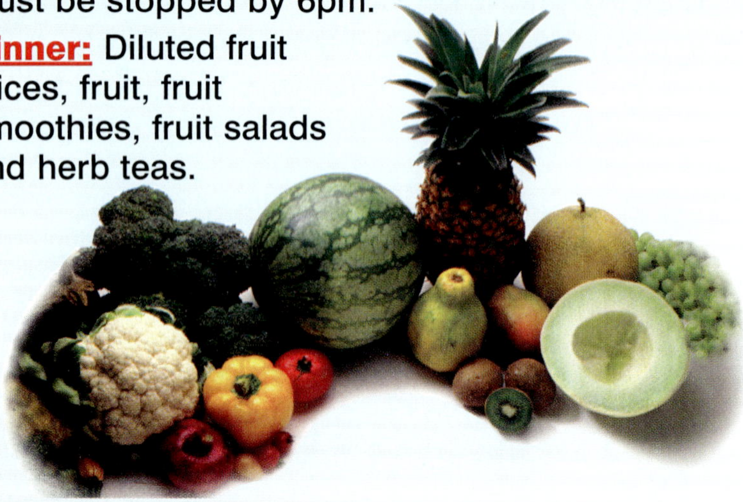

DAY #2, #3, AND #4

Now we begin the 3-day fast. Consume at least 1 gallon (128 ounces) of liquid a day. That's eight 16-ounce servings a day. If you get hungry, DRINK MORE LIQUID!!!

Mornings: Start with water, your morning flush, herbal teas/tonics and your morning SuperFood drink.

Mid-mornings: Diluted fruit juices, herb teas and water until noon.

Afternoons: Diluted vegetable juices, potassium broth, herb teas and water until evening.

Evenings: Diluted fruit juice, herb teas and water in the evening.

DAY #5

Day #5 is the day you will be breaking your fast. Your food program will be the same as day #1. Breaking your fast is a very important part of this program. Chew your food slowly and mix each mouthful with plenty of saliva. Eat until you are satisfied, not full. You can always eat more later if you are still hungry. Chew everything to a liquid pulp.

See Dr. Schulze's Recipes for the Kidney/Bladder Flush Drink on page 43, and Kidney Stone Dissolving Formula on the Next Page

Kidney Stone Dissolving Routine

This routine takes 2 days and can be repeated. Take a stainless steel pot and fill it with 3 quarts (96 ounces) of Fresh Squeezed Organic Apple Juice. Use strong apples that have a lot of organic mallic acid, that make you pucker, not some tasteless politically correct delicious apples that have little or no nutritional or medicinal benefit at all. Add 20 ounces of Fresh Squeezed Organic Citrus Juice, Lemon and Lime half and half is best. Then add 10 ounces of Organic, Raw, Unfiltered Apple Cider Vinegar. Add 1 entire bottle of my Kidney and Bladder Formula and 2 entire packages of my Kidney and Bladder Tea. Let this mixture steep in a warm place for a whole day, stirring every couple of hours for a minute or two. If you have a real serious stone problem, add a few additional ounces of Hydrangea root and a few more ounces of Gravel root to this brew.

To make this Formula stronger, mix all the ingredients in a blender. This will break down and smash all the herbs. Let this sit for 24 hours, then strain through a stainless steel strainer or squeeze through a clean, cotton t-shirt. **The strained formula must now be kept in the refrigerator until it is all consumed.**

DR. SCHULZE'S KIDNEY STONE DISSOLVING FORMULA

- **Gallon Jug**
- **96 ounces Organic, Fresh Squeezed Apple Juice**
- **10 ounces Organic, Fresh Squeezed Lemon Juice**
- **10 ounces Organic, Fresh Squeezed Lime Juice**
- **10 ounces Organic, Raw, Unfiltered Apple Cider Vinegar**
- **One 2 oz. bottle of Dr. Schulze's Kidney/Bladder Formula**
- **Two 4 oz. bags of Dr. Schulze's Kidney/Bladder Herb Tea**

The next day after it has brewed, drink 4 ounces an hour of the liquid. You can even drink an ounce every 15 minutes. Considering that you sleep 8 hours and are up for 16, if you drink 4 ounces every hour that you are awake, you will consume a total of 64 ounces each day which means this brew will last you almost 2 days.

You will also be drinking some distilled water, up to 64 ounces a day. Only distilled water, the ***emptiest*** water, is allowed. Distilled water is so empty, it is like a vacuum, it is the universal solvent especially for unwanted mineral deposits. Just by drinking distilled water on a regular basis you dissolve stones, and prevent new ones from forming, but when added to this routine, you'll have a real winner.

PATIENT CASE HISTORY

I had literally hundreds of patients who came to my clinic with Kidney stones and all of them were able to dissolve them.

I had a man, in his early 30's come to see me from UCLA Hospital where they x-rayed him and found 19 large Kidney stones. One doctor suggested Kidney surgery and the other suggested the sound wave blaster that breaks up the stones. And they hopefully don't get stuck on the way out, OUCH!!!!!

Instead he had heard from a friend of a friend who I helped dissolve their Kidney Stones, so he came to me. I put him on my Kidney Stone Dissolving Routine and then we did it a second time for good measure. Against my advice he returned to the hospital about 2 weeks later for another x-ray where they discovered that his stones were gone, ***VOILA!***

Remember when dissolving any type of stone, Kidney, Gallbladder, whatever, 100 small stones will dissolve faster than 1 large stone, just like a bag of ice cubes will melt faster than a big block of ice. So the program can be repeated as often as needed until all the gravel, or the Rock of Gibraltar is gone.

CHAPTER SIX

THE SOLUTION DR. SCHULZE'S HERBAL FORMULAE

KIDNEY/BLADDER FORMULA

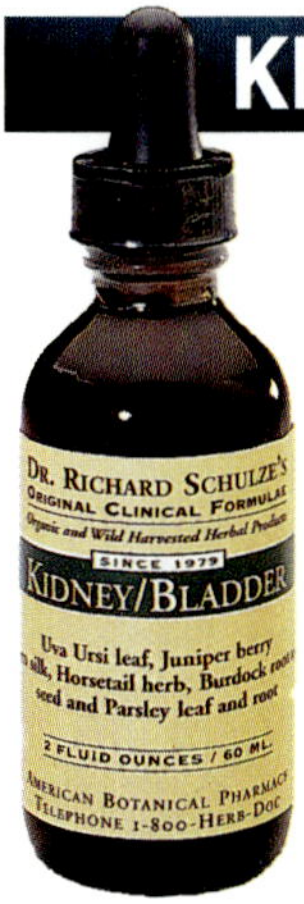

DIURETIC & DISINFECTANT TO THE KIDNEYS, BLADDER AND URINARY SYSTEM.

DR. SCHULZE DESCRIBES HIS K/B FORMULA:

This tonic is both diuretic (increases the flow of urine) and disinfectant (destroys urinary tract infections) to the Kidneys, Bladder, and Urinary System. Although this action has been known and reported since the beginning of recorded herbal medicine, modern medicine has finally filled its medical books documenting this powerful medicinal action.

Whenever I used these formulae in my clinic, they cured every patient with a urinary tract infection, even after antibiotics had failed. It worked 100% of the time. This formula works best if used along with the Kidney/Bladder Tea on the page 52 and the Kidney/Bladder Flush Drink as directed in Chapter 4.

WHAT OUR CUSTOMERS SAY ABOUT K/B FORMULA:

Dear Dr. Schulze,

I have been plagued with reoccurring Kidney and Bladder infections all of my life. I just want to give you a big hug because your Kidney and Bladder Herbal Products and Program did what no medical doctor and no

antibiotic could ever do, which is heal my kidney infection for good! God Bless You.

S.B. Los Angeles, CA

METABOLIC ACTION AND BOTANICAL CHEMISTRY:

Uva Ursi leaf contains powerful phytochemicals such as volatile oils, arbutin, quercetin, and mallic and gallic acids. Arbutin is highly antibacterial and destroys bacteria and fungus that infect the urinary system such as E. coli, Candida albicans, Staphylococcus, etc. One of the ways arbutin does this is by releasing aglycone hydroquinone and other phytochemicals into the urine. Quercetin is a capillary protectant, protecting the literally trillions of capillaries existing as part of the delicate kidney filtering system. Mallic and Gallic acids, the same as found in apples and apple cider vinegar, have long been used for kidney and bladder infections.

All of the other herbs in this formula contain phytochemicals that are either diuretic, anti-microbial or anti-inflammatory to the entire urinary system.

BOTANICAL INGREDIENTS:

Uva Ursi leaf, Arctostaphylos uva ursi, Juniper berries, Juniperus communis, Corn silk, Zea mays, Horsetail herb, Equisetum arvense, Burdock root and seed, Arctium lappa, Parsley leaf and root, Petroselinum crispum, Pipsissewa leaf, Chimaphilla umbellata and Goldenrod flower tops, Solidago virgaurea.

DOSAGE:

1-2 droppersful (30-60 drops) in a few ounces of water 3 to 4 times daily, depending on the diuretic action needed or the seriousness of the infection. Best results are obtained if used for 10 days or until the 2 ounce bottle is finished.

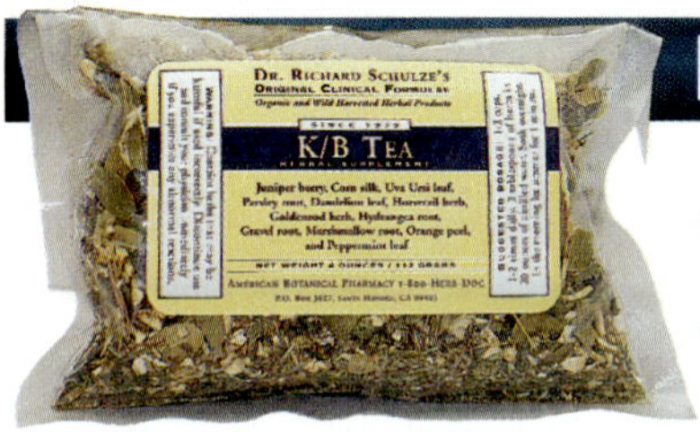

KIDNEY/BLADDER TEA

DIURETIC, DISINFECTANT AND DISSOLVENT

DESCRIBES THE K/B TEA:

A mild-tasting but powerfully effective tea. It is both diuretic and antiseptic to the entire urinary tract, but it also soothes urinary tract inflammation and also dissolves kidney stones and renal gravel.

This formula has all the actions of the Kidney/Bladder Formula, though slightly milder, but has additional herbs for reducing inflammation in the urinary tract and also for dissolving kidney stones and renal calculi.

WHAT OUR CUSTOMERS SAY ABOUT K/B TEA:

I can't believe something that tastes so mild could be so powerful and heal my long term bladder infection and cystitis.

U.F. Santa Monica, CA

METABOLIC ACTION AND BOTANICAL CHEMISTRY:

The herbs in this formula have the identical action as the Kidney and Bladder Formula with the addition of **Hydrangea root** and **Gravel root** which are specifics for dissolving kidney stones and renal calculi.

Juniper berries are by far my favorite Kidney and Bladder herb. I used them in every clinical Kidney and Bladder Formula I ever made. I found them to be the diuretic herb that always worked, and a urinary disinfectant that worked even on the most stubborn cases. I believe this is due to their wonderful essential and volatile oils. They worked miracles in my clinic, but are not officially recognized for any of the above uses, but Uva Ursi is.

BOTANICAL INGREDIENTS:

Juniper berries, *Juniperus communis,* **Corn silk,** *Zea mays,* **Uva Ursi leaves,** *Arctostaphylos uva ursi,* **Parsley root and leaf,** *Petroselinum crispum,* **Carrot tops,** *Daucus carota,* **Dandelion leaf,** *Taraxacum officinale,* **Horsetail herb,** *Equisetum arvense,* **Goldenrod flower tops,** *Solidago virgaurea,* **Hydrangea root,** *Hydrangea arboresens,* **Gravel root,** *Eupatorium purpureum,* **Marshmallow root,** *Althaea officinalis,* **Orange peel,** *Citrus species,* **and Peppermint leaf,** *Mentha piperita.*

DOSAGE:

2 cups three times daily.

Directions to start the tea:

Put 6 tablespoons of this tea into 60 ounces of distilled water. Be sure to use only stainless steel or glass cookware. Let the tea sit in the water overnight. In the morning, heat it to a boil, reduce heat, and let simmer for 1 minute. Strain the herbs; do not discard them. Let the tea cool a bit, but use it hot. This will give you enough tea to drink 2 cups 3 times during the day. If you are planning to drink the tea for more than 1 day, then after the first day put the used herbs back into the pot, adding 3 tablespoons of fresh herbs and 60 ounces of distilled water. Let sit overnight and repeat the whole process. Keep adding new herbs to the old ones for three days, then discard all herbs and start over.

D-TOX FORMULA

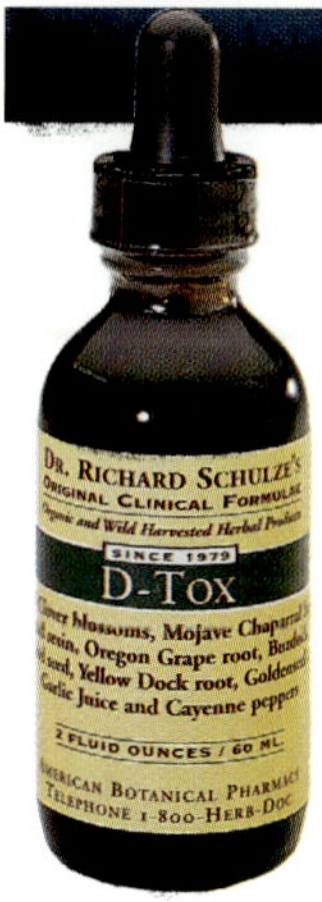

A VERY POWERFUL BLOOD AND LYMPH CLEANSING FORMULA THAT SCRUBS THE ACCUMULATED TOXINS AND POISONS OUT OF THE BODY.

DR. SCHULZE DESCRIBES THE D-TOX FORMULA:

Some of the botanicals in this politically incorrect herbal formula have been vigorously attacked by our federal government and medical groups during the past century, some within the past 10 years. These gifts from God have created everything from Senate hearings, witch hunts and raids led by government agencies and vicious AMA attacks to having American Herbalists and Naturopathic Physicians thrown in jail and even exiled from the country. What are they so afraid of? I'd say that speaks for itself. Some of these herbs have been illegal to use, like Chaparral, which was outlawed for almost 5 years. Suppliers stopped selling it and herbalists sucked-up politically. I instead harvested my own in the California deserts and continued to use it. After all, in my clinic, potent healing ability dictated which herbs I put in my formulations and used with my patients, NOT politics. How could I look a patient in the eye who was suffering and tell them that I know what helps, but legally I can't sell it to you? Because I continued to use this herb during its prohibition, this became just one of the reasons my clinic was shut down. Other botanicals in the formula are highly discouraged by medical doctors like Lobelia seed, Poke root, even Red Clover Blossoms. **Consequently, many herbalists, myself included, have been arrested and incarcerated for even discussing the benefits of these**

types of herbs because of their association with treating cancer and chronic disease. Having said all of this I must tell you that the herbs in this formula are classic and traditional blood and lymph cleansing tonics and the ones that I used successfully for many years in my clinic. I would have EVERY patient in my clinic do my 5-Day Cleansing and Detoxification Program and consume one entire bottle of this formula within a week's time.

This formula is based on the famous Hoxey Formula, Dr. Christopher's Red Clover Combination (both herbalists were arrested on numerous occasions for these formulations) and many similar powerful Alternative (blood cleansing) formula from around the world. These herbs are used in herbal medical clinics worldwide for scrubbing the accumulated toxins and poisons out of the body's blood, fat and cells and also heralded for their efficacy.

WHAT OUR CUSTOMERS SAY ABOUT D-TOX FORMULA:

(No Comment) By law we cannot print what our customers say about this formula.

METABOLIC ACTION AND BOTANICAL CHEMISTRY:

The following is common knowledge from highly respected and accepted medical text. According to pharmacology manuals, Chaparral contains Nordihydroguaiaretic acid. According to the Merck Index, one of the most respected medical chemical books in the world, this acid from chaparral is listed as an anti-oxidant with a Therapeutic Category as an Anti-neoplastic. According to Taber's Cyclopedic Medical Dictionary, an Anti-neoplastic is "an agent that Prevents the development, growth and proliferation of malignant cells."

BOTANICAL INGREDIENTS:

Red Clover blossoms, *Trifolium pratense,* **Mojave Chaparral herb & resin,** *Larrea californica,* **Oregon Grape root,** *Berberis aquifolium,* **Burdock root & seed,** *Arctium lappa,* **Yellow Dock root,** *Rumex crispus,* **Goldenseal root,** *Hydrastis canadensis,* **Garlic juice,** *Allium sativum,* **Cayenne peppers,** *Capsicum annuum,* **Poke root,** *Phytolacca Bloodroot,* **and Lobelia seeds,** *Lobelia inflata.*

DOSAGE:

The herbs in this formula are extremely strong in taste. Dilute in a few ounces of fresh juice, grape works the best. **For general use:** 2 droppersful (60 drops) 3 to 4 times a day for a week. You must consume the entire bottle during the 5-Day Cleansing Program or as described in the Incurables Program. Drink 64-128 ounces of liquid a day while taking this formula.

CHAPTER SEVEN

FINAL THOUGHTS

When building a house you need lots of different tools. To start you need large powerful bulldozers to grade the site level and dig the trenches for the foundation. Then you need concrete mixers, sledge hammers, big heavy framing hammers, table saws and hand held power tools to build the frame of the house. Finally for the finish work you need more delicate tools like small screwdrivers, pliers, small finish hammers, sandpaper and paint brushes.

In my clinic I created numerous Natural Healing and Herbal tools, some small tools, some medium tools and some real BIG and STRONG tools. In my clinic I learned the importance of picking the right tool for the job and I learned the importance of having a variety of tools. I needed my big powerful Natural Healing Routines and Herbal Medicine tools for the big jobs (like my Incurables Program and my Detoxification Tonic), to help my patients heal their serious and life-threatening diseases. I also needed an assortment of finishing and maintenance tools (like my 5-Day Detoxification and Cleansing Program and my SuperFood) to help my patients build healthy and strong bodies, and to keep them healthy for years to come.

Since my clinic is closed, and I'm not there to personally guide you through your Natural Healing Programs, when in doubt do them more intensely and for a longer period of time. Remember, the people who don't get well using Natural Healing, **don't get well** because they didn't do enough... not because they did too much.

➤ *You've READ about it...*

Hear what somebody else says:

Dear Dr. Schulze,
I was diagnosed with a urinary infection and my doctor suggested I take an antibiotic. There my horror began. Some of the antibiotics I could not tolerate and I remember my long, horrible nights when I was on my knees above the bathroom bowl. I suffered alot. By luck, I heard of your methods and ideas. I started to do what you advised and within a few months I was free of infection and I've stayed disease free ever since. I used many of your recipes and recommendations with great success. I have two juice machines and my medical cabinet is filled with a real staff like your Kidney Formula, Echinacea, Deep Tissue, etc.
Sincerely,
V.V. Auburn, AL

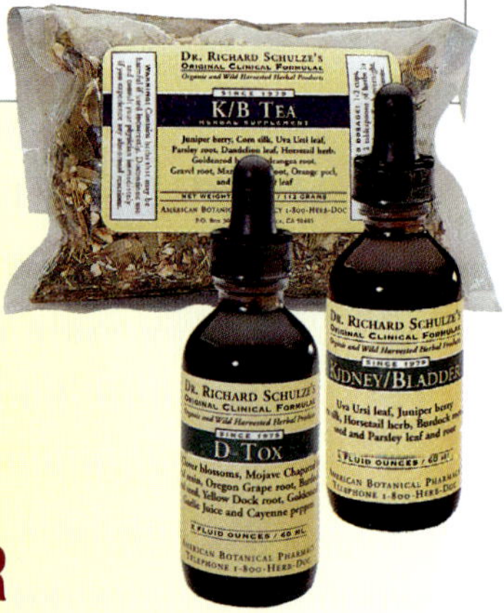

➤ *NOW is the time to*

CLEANSE YOUR Kidneys & Bladder with

Dr. Schulze's Famous
5-DAY KIDNEY/BLADDER Cleansing and Detoxification Program along with his KIDNEY/BLADDER FLUSH DRINK.

EASY, SIMPLE and FAST!

DR. RICHARD SCHULZE'S

AMERICAN BOTANICAL PHARMACY

ORIGINAL CLINICAL HERBAL FORMULAE SINCE 1979

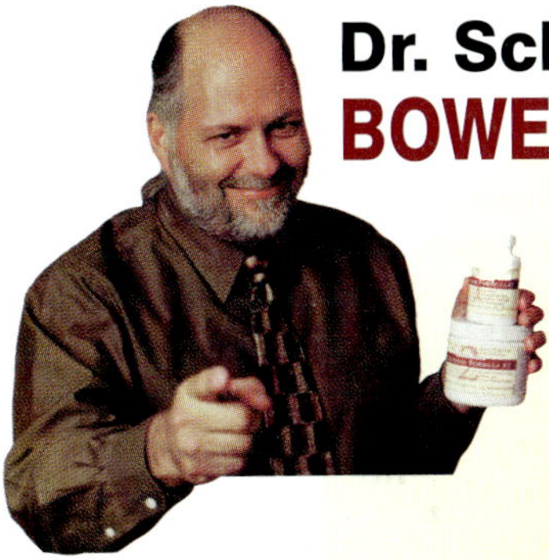

Dr. Schulze's Famous BOWEL DETOXIFICATION Program

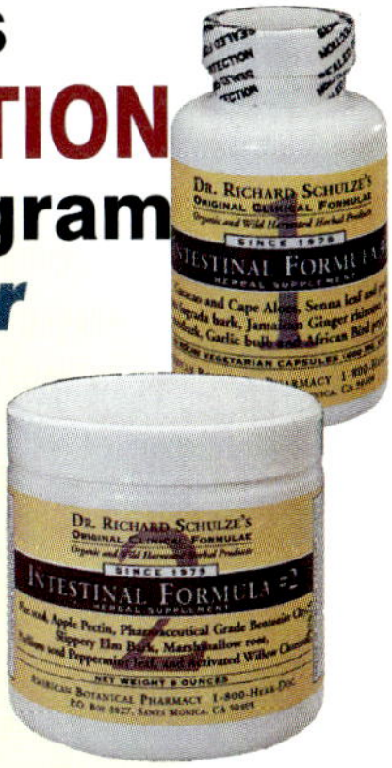

"Cleansing your Colon is the FIRST step to better health."

More than 100,000 people worldwide have used this program to **ELIMINATE** constipation, **CLEANSE** their colon, **DETOXIFY** their body, and **HEAL** and **PREVENT** Colon Disease.

After doing this Program, be prepared to call all your friends and tell them you just had the BEST BOWEL MOVEMENT OF YOUR LIFE!

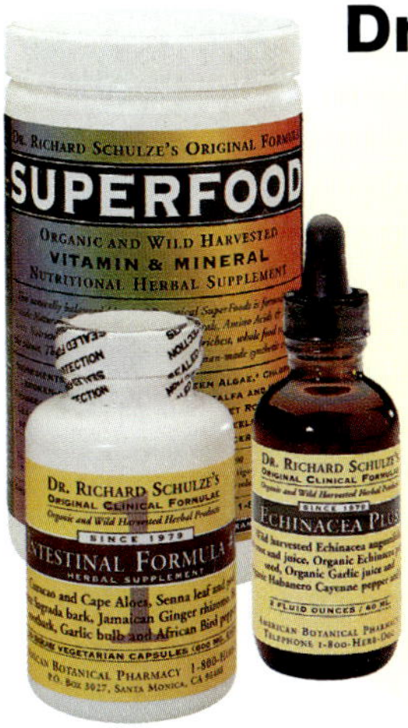

Dr. Schulze's Famous "WHERE DO I START?" Program

"This program is the place to START if you don't know what to do! If you want Better Health and More Energy, but you want it CHEAP, only have 2 MINUTES and it must be EASY! Then this program is for you because all YOU have to do is swallow, and I guarantee the Results!"

- Dr. Richard Schulze

ASK for YOUR FREE CATALOG!

TO ORDER CALL

1-800-HERBDOC

IT'S THAT SIMPLE!

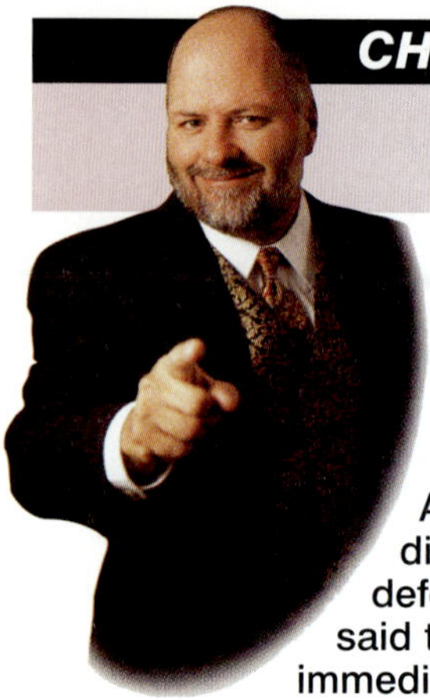

CHAPTER TEN

About the AUTHOR

Personal Healing When he was only 11 years old, his father died in his arms from a massive heart attack. At 14, his mother died of a heart attack. They were both only 55 years old.

At age 16 after a year of ill health, he was diagnosed by medical doctors with a genetic heart deformity and deformed heart valves. The doctors said that unless he underwent open heart surgery immediately, he would be dead by the age of 20. This is because his weak deformed heart couldn't supply sufficient blood to an adult body.

He declined to have the surgery and instead made it his mission to discover alternative ways to heal his heart. After three years of numerous intensive natural healing programs and herbal formulae, he was given a clean bill of health by the very surprised medical doctors. His heart was healed. After curing himself of this so-called "incurable" disease, through changes in his lifestyle and NO surgery, he then set out on a mission to help others. He enrolled himself into Naturopathic and Herbal College.

Education and Credentials Dr. Schulze studied with the famous European Naturopath, Paavo Airola. He trained and then served an internship with the famous natural healer Dr. Bernard Jensen. He also studied and apprenticed with "America's greatest clinical herbalist", the late Dr. John Christopher, graduating to teach alongside him until his death. Besides having a Doctorate in Herbology and a Doctorate in Natural Medicine and three degrees in Iridology, he is certified in eight different styles of Body Therapy and holds three black belts in the Martial Arts.

Clinical Experience In the early 1970's he opened his first Natural Healing Clinic in New York, and later in Southern California. He operated his natural healing clinic in America for almost 20 years, until his clinic was shut down. During this same time he also managed and directed other Natural Healing Clinics in Europe and Asia. In his two decades of practice he treated thousands of patients. In his second decade of clinical practice, he became famous for his intensive natural healing programs and his powerful herbal formulae.

His natural therapy programs and herbal formulae are now used in clinics all over the world and have assisted an estimated hundred thousand people to create healing miracles and regain their health.

He is considered an innovator, a purist, even an extremist by many of his colleagues, but to his patients he was considered a life saver. Dr. Schulze always said, ***"While Alternative doctors are pussy footing***

around trying to heal degenerative disease with aromatherapy and purple candles, the medical doctors are sharpening their knives, saws and drills, boiling down their chemotherapy and fine tuning their radiation beams. At least medical doctors know how to treat killer diseases, aggressively and with intensity." In his clinic he was famous for his powerful and extreme natural healing programs and his potent clinical herbal formulae. He often said, ***"I tried to kill my patients with the juicer, I tried to poison them with overdoses of strong herbal tonics, I tried to drown them in hydrotherapy, but the only thing that happened is that they got well. All the people I see dying and not recovering who are being treated with alternative medicine, are dying because they aren't doing enough. They need a natural healing blitz, turn the volume all the way up, and create a 24 hour a day natural healing lifestyle."***

Dr. Schulze dared to pioneer new techniques and therapies which went far beyond what most people thought possible with Alternative medicine. The outcome of his work has been the achievement of miraculous and unprecedented results. His herbal formulae and 30-Day Cleansing and Detoxification "Incurables" Program are used in clinics worldwide to help people heal themselves from degenerative diseases such as Heart Disease, Cancer, Arthritis and AIDS. The positive results have caused reverberations in both the natural and medical communities.

A Passionate, Electrifying Teacher Dr. Schulze assisted and taught for the late Dr. John Christopher. After Dr. Christopher's death, Dr. Schulze continued to teach at his school for over 12 years. He has served as the Director of The College of Herbology and Natural Healing in the United Kingdom for 11 years and is also Co-Director of The Osho School for Naturopathic Medicine in England, France and Spain. Dr. Schulze has taught and lectured at numerous universities, including Cambridge and Oxford Universities in England, Trinity Medical College in Ireland, Omega Institute in New York, Cortijo Romero in Spain and other natural therapy and herbal institutes worldwide. He has been the guest speaker at numerous churches and also on numerous radio and television shows. He is loved for his intensity, passion, dedication to students, sense of humor, creativity, and his exciting, enthusiastic and evangelistic teaching style. He is mostly recognized for his unequaled understanding of natural healing. He continues to teach throughout the United States and Europe.

American Botanical Pharmacy After 15 years of manufacturing his own herbal formulations in his clinic, Dr. Schulze opened American Botanical Pharmacy in 1994 which manufactures and sells his industrial-strength, pharmaceutical grade botanical extracts.

Dr. Schulze continues his healing mission today through his daily work to reveal the truth about the unlimited healing power of our bodies. He is also a leader in exposing fraud in medical, pharmaceutical and even herbal industries. He records numerous audio and video tapes, writes many books and booklets and publishes his free newsletters, all through Natural Healing Publications.

Dr. Schulze's EDUCATIONAL STARTER KIT

"IF YOU WANT TO KNOW WHERE TO GET STARTED... IT'S HERE!"

THIS SPECIAL DEAL GIVES YOU EVERYTHING YOU NEED TO GET STARTED TODAY!

GET *BOTH* FOR ONLY $20.00
Reg. Price $26.00
You Save 23%

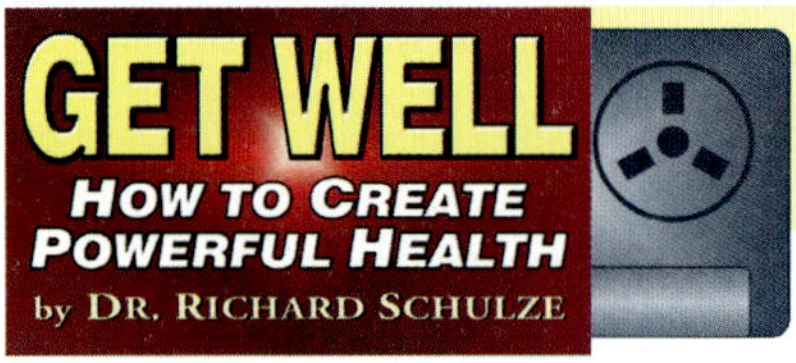

GET WELL
HOW TO CREATE POWERFUL HEALTH

90-minute audio tape
Reg. Price $10.00

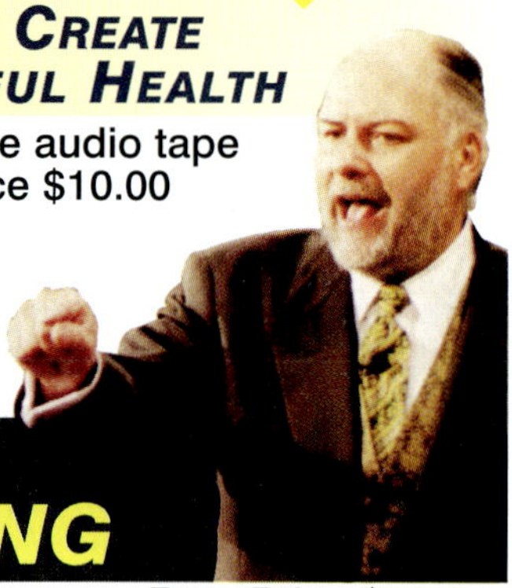

"The ABSOLUTE BEST introduction to Natural Healing you will ever find!"

COMMON SENSE HEALTH and HEALING

200 pages Reg. Price $16.00

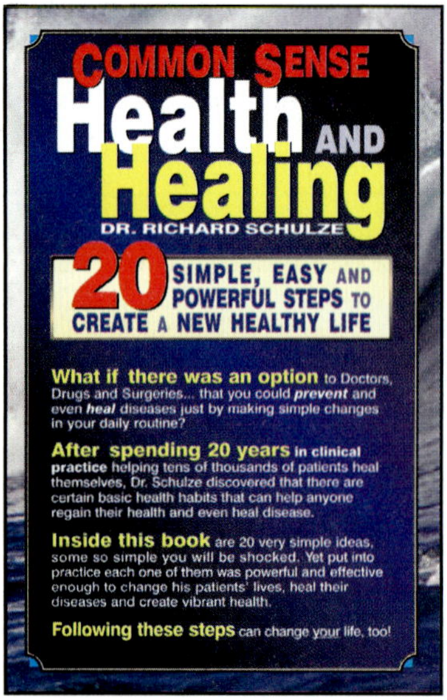

What if there was an option to Doctors, Drugs and Surgeries... that you could ***prevent*** and even ***heal*** diseases just by making simple changes in your daily routine?

After spending 20 years in clinical practice helping tens of thousands of patients heal themselves, Dr. Schulze discovered that there are certain basic health habits that can help anyone regain their health and even heal disease.

Inside this book are 20 very simple ideas, some so simple you will be shocked. Yet put into practice each one of them was powerful and effective enough to change his patients' lives, heal their diseases and create vibrant health. ***Following these steps*** can ***change your life!***

Additional NATURAL HEALING Resources from DR. SCHULZE

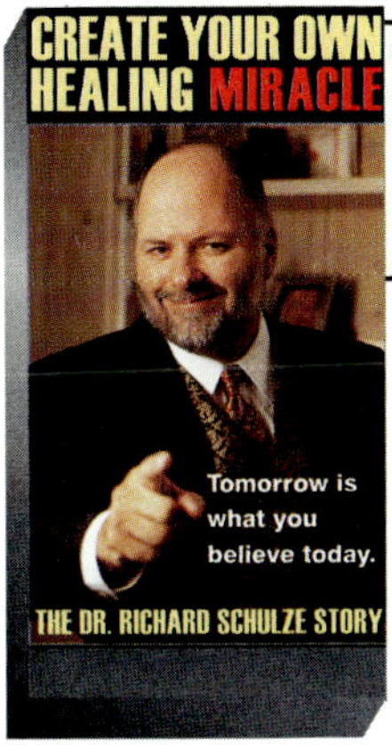

CREATE YOUR OWN HEALING MIRACLE
THE DR. RICHARD SCHULZE STORY

In this powerful 2 HOUR VIDEO Dr. Schulze tells how he healed himself of a killer heart disease, 4th degree burns, and a crippling knee injury. The doctors said he would be dead by age 20 without open heart surgery, never grow his skin back without multiple skin graft operations, and never walk again without extensive knee surgery. Watch how and why he proved them all wrong.

This tape includes 45 minutes of live, unsolicited testimonials by people who were told that without surgery, drugs, chemotherapy or radiation they would be sick the rest of their lives. Some were even sent home to die. These people knew the awesome healing power of Dr. Schulze's programs first hand, because, against all odds, they created their own HEALING MIRACLES. This video will inspire you to take control of your health and CREATE ***YOUR OWN*** PERSONAL HEALING MIRACLE. 2 hour video $15.00

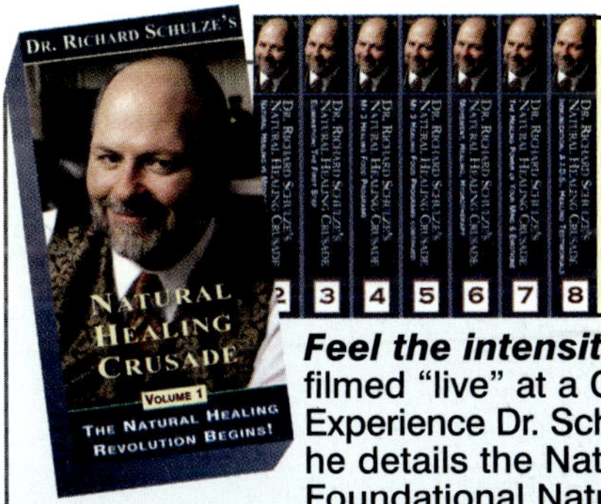

DR. RICHARD SCHULZE'S NATURAL HEALING CRUSADE
VIDEO COLLECTION

Feel the intensity of Dr. Schulze's enthusiasm filmed "live" at a California Natural Healing Crusade! Experience Dr. Schulze's raw passion, wit and wisdom as he details the Natural Healing Power in ALL of his Foundational Natural Healing programs. ***It's like having him in your own living room!*** In this video series, he gives you the same step-by-step instructions he gave to every one of his patients in his clinic for over 20 years.

IN THIS 8-PART VIDEO SERIES DR. SCHULZE COVERS:

- **The Foundation of Natural Healing**
- **Blockage: The Cause of all Disease**
- **Elimination: The First Step**
- **Dr. Schulze's 3 Healing Food Programs**
- **Movement, Circulation, Hydrotherapy**
- **The Healing Power of Your Mind and Emotions**
- **Healing Testimonials**

8 video series
$98.00

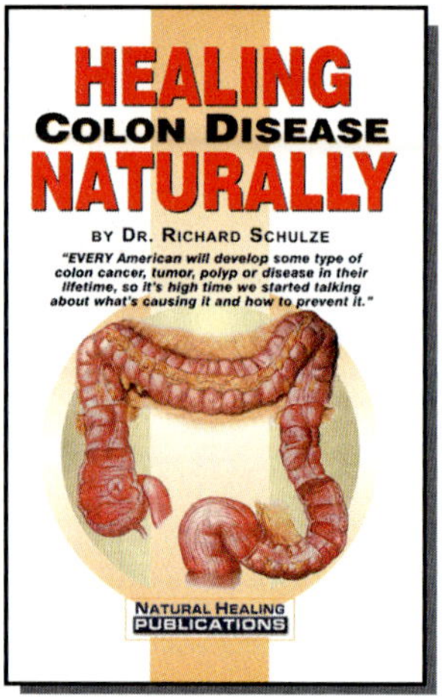

64 pages $7.00

HEALING COLON DISEASE NATURALLY

"NEVER, NEVER, NEVER UNDERESTIMATE THE HEALING POWER OF COLON CLEANSING."

Inside this book you will clearly see that the real cause behind the majority of sickness and disease in America is the retention and storage of toxic, poisonous waste in our colon and the infrequency of it emptying. I will show you how cleansing your colon will make the biggest healing difference in your life, help you to heal any disease and sickness and create powerful lasting health and vitality.

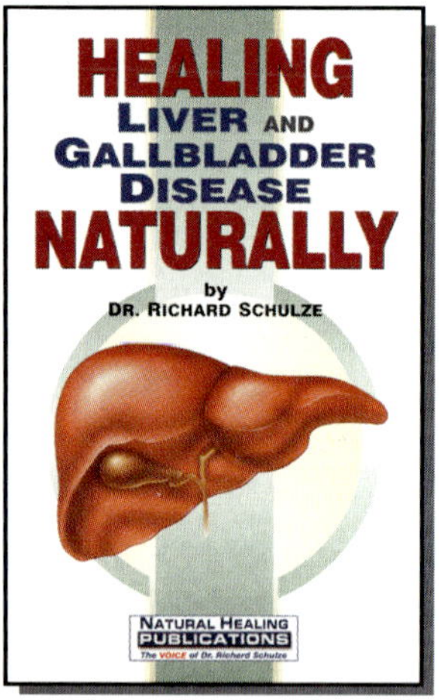

64 pages $7.00

HEALING LIVER AND GALLBLADDER DISEASE NATURALLY

"Your LIVER Cleans Your Blood!"

Heart disease, cancer – most ALL diseases – develop months, even years after your liver failed to keep your blood clean.

What if you could add 10 years to your life by just doing a simple cleanse a few days a year? Dr. Schulze shows you how cleansing and detoxifying your Liver and Gallbladder will make the biggest healing difference in your life!

GET A FREE Catalog OF ALL DR. SCHULZE'S NATURAL HEALING BOOKS, DVD'S/VIDEOS AND AUDIO TAPES.

JUST CALL NATURAL HEALING PUBLICATIONS

1-877-TEACH ME (832-2463)